Cytologic Detection of Urothelial Lesions

IN CYTOPATHOLOGY SERIES

Dorothy L. Rosenthal, MD, FIAC, Series Editor

Editorial Board:
  Syed Z. Ali, MD
  Douglas P. Clark, MD
  Yener S. Erozan, MD

---

1. D.P. Clark and W.C. Faquin: Thyroid Cytopathology. 2005
ISBN 0-387-23304-0
2. D.L. Rosenthal and S.S. Raab: Cytologic Detection of Urothelial Lesions. 2005
ISBN 0-387-23945-6

Dorothy L. Rosenthal, MD, FIAC

The Johns Hopkins University School of Medicine
Baltimore, Maryland

Stephen S. Raab, MD

University of Pittsburgh Medical Center
Pittsburgh, Pennsylvania

Cytologic Detection of Urothelial Lesions

With 131 Illustrations in Full Color

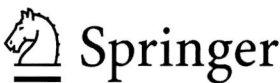

Dorothy L. Rosenthal, M.D., FIAC
Professor of Pathology, Oncology, and Gynecology/Obstetrics
The Johns Hopkins School of Medicine
Baltimore, MD 21287
USA

Stephen S. Raab, M.D.
Professor of Pathology
Chief of Pathology, UPMC Shadyside
University of Pittsburgh Medical Center
Pittsburgh, PA 15213
USA

Library of Congress Cataloging-in-Publication Data
Rosenthal, Dorothy L.
　　Cytologic detection of urothelial lesions / Dorothy L. Rosenthal
　and Stephen S. Raab.
　　　p.　cm. – (Essentials in cytopathology series ; v. 2)
　Includes bibliographical references and index.
　ISBN 0-387-23945-6 (alk. paper) – 0-387-23947-2 (e-ISBN)
　1. Urinary organs—Diseases—Cytodiagnosis.　I. Raab, Stephen S.
II. Title.　III. Series.
　RC901.R67 2006
　616.6'07582—dc22　　　　　　　　　　　　　　　　2004061417

ISBN-10: 0-387-23945-6　　　　　e-ISBN: 0-387-23947-2
ISBN-13: 978-0387-23945-3　　　　Printed on acid-free paper.

© 2006 Springer Science+Business Media, Inc.
All rights reserved. This work may not be translated or copied in whole or in part without the written permission of the publisher (Springer Science+Business Media, Inc., 233 Spring Street, New York, NY 10013, USA), except for brief excerpts in connection with reviews or scholarly analysis. Use in connection with any form of information storage and retrieval, electronic adaptation, computer software, or by similar or dissimilar methodology now known or hereafter developed is forbidden. The use in this publication of trade names, trademarks, service marks and similar terms, even if they are not identified as such, is not to be taken as an expression of opinion as to whether or not they are subject to proprietary rights.

While the advice and information in this book are believed to be true and accurate at the date of going to press, neither the authors nor the editors nor the publisher can accept any legal responsibility for any errors or omissions that may be made. The publisher makes no warranty, express or implied, with respect to the material contained herein.

Printed in China　　(TB/EVB)

9　8　7　6　5　4　3　2　1

springeronline.com

*To our families and friends for their love and support,
and to the legacy of the late George L. Wied, M.D., FIAC.*

Foreword

Dr. Rosenthal and Dr. Raab correctly place urinary cytology in the backwater of the field, noting the difficulties many of us encounter when assessing urinary specimens or washes of the urinary tract. For a variety of reasons, these specimens are saved for the end of the day, cause the most trouble and frustration, and are the least successful from the standpoint of the pathologist, the urologist, or the patient.

This book represents, in keeping with the philosophy behind the series, *Essentials in Cytopathology*, a systematic description of microscopic findings in urinary specimens, whether normal, reactive, or neoplastic, accompanied by an extensive collection of photomicrographs (in color) illustrative of the full range of lesions. Drawing upon their personal collections and the diagnostic resources of several major cytologic laboratories, they have assembled examples of the common diagnostic entities in the field plus an assortment of confounding circumstances, which contribute to the difficulties presented by urinary specimens. Handy tables accompany the photographs, offering help where needed. This is particularly relevant because the subtlety of urinary cytology defies the dependable diagnostic categorization obtained with samples from other sites.

Reading this book set me to thinking about the evolution of texts in pathology from exhaustive narratives about visual concepts accompanied by relatively few black and white photographs or drawings in black and white or rarely with added color. Many of us can recall when colored photomicrographs were not available and when they became available but were not affordable. Now, it is unusual to find black and white photographs in medical texts, electron micrographs aside. Young physicians, having extensive experience with digital cameras and computers with Photoshop, will feel comfortable with this illustrated book whether beginning their studies in cytology or reviewing urinary cytology in preparation for their board examinations. Even experienced cytotechnologists and cytopathologists may find the illustrations and guidelines useful in the murky waters of urinary cytology, thanks to Dr. Rosenthal and Dr. Raab.

Jerry Waisman
February 20, 2005

Series Preface

The subspecialty of cytopathology is 60 years old and has become established as a solid and reliable discipline in medicine. As expected, cytopathology literature has expanded in a remarkably short period of time, from a few textbooks prior to the 1980s to a current library of texts and journals devoted exclusively to cytomorphology that is substantial. *Essentials in Cytopathology* does not presume to replace any of the distinguished textbooks in Cytopathology. Instead, the series will publish generously illustrated and user-friendly guides for both pathologists and clinicians.

Building on the amazing success of *The Bethesda System for Reporting Cervical Cytology*, now in its second edition, the series will utilize a similar format including minimal text, tabular criteria and superb illustrations based on real-life specimens. *Essentials in Cytopathology* will, at times, deviate from the classic organization of pathology texts. The logic of decision trees, elimination of unlikely choices and narrowing of differential diagnosis via a pragmatic approach based on morphologic criteria will be some of the strategies used to illustrate principles and practice in Cytopathology.

Most of the authors for *Essentials in Cytopathology* are faculty members in The Johns Hopkins University School of Medicine, Department of Pathology, Division of Cytopathology. They bring to each volume the legacy of John K. Frost and the collective experience of a preeminent cytopathology service. The archives at Hopkins are meticulously catalogued and form the framework for text and illustrations. Authors from other institutions have been selected on the basis of their national reputations, experience and enthusiasm for cytopathology. They bring to the series complementary viewpoints and enlarge the scope of materials contained in the photographs.

The editor and authors are indebted to our students, past and future, who challenge and motivate us to become the best that we possibly can be. We share that experience with you through these pages, and hope that you will learn from them as we have from those who have come before us. We would be remiss if we did not pay tribute to our professional colleagues, the cytotechnologists and preparatory technicians who lovingly care for the specimens that our clinical colleagues send to us.

And finally, we cannot emphasize enough throughout these volumes the importance of collaboration with the patient care team. Every specimen comes to us as a question begging an answer. Without input from the clinicians, complete patient history, results of imaging studies and other ancillary tests, we cannot perform optimally. It is our responsibility to educate our clinicians about their role in our interpretation, and for us to integrate as much information as we can gather into our final diagnosis, even if the answer at first seems obvious.

We hope you will find this series useful and welcome your feedback as you place these handbooks by your microscopes, and into your bookbags.

Dorothy L. Rosenthal, M.D., FIAC
Baltimore Maryland
drosenthal@jhmi.edu

July 15, 2004

Contents

Foreword vii
Series Preface ix

Cytologic Detection of Urothelial Lesions 1
    Introduction 1
    Background...................................... 2

1 Normal Morphology 5
    Anatomic Considerations 5
    Normal Urothelial Histology and Cytology 5

2 Diagnostic Categories 19
    Formatting the Report 19
    Morphologic Differences Dependent on Method
    of Sample Collection............................ 20
    Benign Cellular Changes—Normal/Reactive 21
    Benign Non-epithelial Elements 22
    Atypical Urothelial Cells Indeterminate
    for Neoplasia 22

3 Grading Urothelial Neoplasms (Transitional Cell
   Carcinoma, TCC)................................. 57
    Terminology, Historic 57
    Terminology used in this Handbook 58
    Low Grade Urothelial Tumors (Grade I, Papilloma,
    Papillary Urothelial Neoplasm of Low
    Malignant Potential) 60

	Low Grade Urothelial Carcinoma (Grade II)	60
	High Grade Urothelial Carcinoma	62
4	Special Circumstances	121
	Ileal Loop or Neo-bladder	121
	Drug-Induced Cytologic Atypias	122
	Radiation-Induced Atypia	124
	Lithiasis	124
5	Unusual Lesions	149
	Lesions Arising in the Bladder	149
	Lesions Arising in the Kidney	149
	Metastases to the Urinary Tract	150
6	Performance Characteristics of Urinary Cytology	165
	Correlation Between Cytology and Histology	165
	Diagnostic Yield of Urinary Cytology	166
7	Specimen Collection and Processing	169
	Collection	169
	Processing	170
Index		175

Note: All figures are stained by the Papanicolaou method unless otherwise stated. H & E is hematoxylin and eosin stain.

Cytologic Detection of Urothelial Lesions

Introduction

This second volume in the Springer-Verlag series, Essentials in Cytopathology, addresses a very difficult and often frustrating area of cytodiagnosis. Unlike gynecological cytology, urinary tract cytologic testing is not intended for the general population. Symptomatic patients, usually hematuria, or those who are at risk for bladder cancer are suitable candidates for morphologic examination of their urine.

The intent of the authors is to present a simple approach to dealing with cellular samples from the urinary tract. Rather than attempting to diagnose the lowest grade lesions as definitive entities, we have placed them in an indeterminate category, along with reactive/atypical changes to infection and therapy. Thus, the clinician is notified that the sample is not normal, but is not forced to "find the lesion". On the other hand, we emphasize the importance of identifying the high grade lesions, as these are life threatening to the patient, and demand careful and directed management to control or eradicate the tumor(s). The need for frequent surveillance of the patient with high grade urothelial carcinoma creates a long term partnership between the cytopathologist and the urologic oncologist. We emphasize the importance of direct and clear communication between the partners since the patient becomes a lifetime candidate for recurrent or new urothelial lesions.

Background

In the U.S., an estimated 56,500 new cases of bladder cancer are detected annually, with approximately 12,600 deaths. These figures may seem insignificant when compared with the incidence and death rates of carcinoma of the lung (169,400 new cases, 154,900 deaths). What is significant is the biologic behavior of most urothelial lesions of the urinary tract, including the ureters and renal pelves. Generally speaking, 5-year survival rates encompass too short a time to tell the full natural history of these tumors, which can easily span 15–20 years. This long survival rate can be attributed to effective chemotherapy and good patient management, but also to the often indolent nature of this unique neoplasm. Although 70% of bladder tumors are superficial or only minimally invasive, and theoretically curable, 50–70% of these patients will have "recurrent" or new tumors, up to a third of which are of higher grade and/or stage. The remaining 30% initially present with muscle invasion or distant metastases.

Synchronous or metachronous tumors may arise in the urothelium of the urinary tract, and can vary in stage and grade when they occur simultaneously. Thus, the clinician and patient are faced with a long-term commitment to control an unpredictable neoplastic process. Obliteration of a low grade tumor in one site provides no guarantee that another tumor, perhaps of higher grade, will not occur in another area.

Cytology plays an important role in the management of these patients. Cystoscopy can visualize and locate papillary lesions of the urinary bladder for biopsy, but lesions of the urethra, ureters, and renal pelves are not as accessible. Radiographic demonstration of a "filling defect" can provide only putative evidence that a tumor is present. Therefore, urinary cytology may be relied upon to indicate if a neoplasm is actually present. The decision to remove a kidney because of suspected ureteral or calyceal tumors or divert the collecting system into an ileal loop or neo-bladder based on cytologic findings places a grave burden of responsibility upon cytologists.

Thus, in order to establish criteria for diagnosing low grade urothelial lesions in the upper urinary tract (ureters and renal pelves) the cytologist must refine diagnostic criteria to distinguish the low grade papillary lesions from benign/reactive atypias. By comparing cytologic specimens derived from bladders that contain histologically proven low grade neoplasms, the cytologist can apply the same criteria to the diagnosis of upper tract lesions, even though the "normal" epithelium has more atypia in the upper tract than the bladder. However, most of the upper tract low grade lesions will not shed diagnostic material unless the sample is obtained after vigorous washing (barbatage).

Although all types of urinary tract lesions, benign and malignant, can be diagnosed theoretically by cytology, only the most common diagnostic problems will be addressed herein. The ambitious student is referred to the referenced works for a more complete discussion. One of the most important factors in becoming proficient in urinary cytology is to effectively communicate with the urologists who submit cytologic specimens. A lesion of the upper tract should never be diagnosed unless the radiographic findings are reviewed with the urologist and the cytologic findings are considered in light of available evidence. Such close collaboration will not only corroborate the cytologic diagnosis, but will provide the urologist with an understanding of the difficulties and problems involved in rendering a reasonable diagnosis. The overwhelming majority of low grade tumors are not life threatening, allowing time for repeat studies to follow the lesion's development and confirm initial impressions.

Suggested Reading

Jemal A, Tiwari RC, Taylor M, Ghafoor A, Samuels A, Ward E, Feuer EJ, Thun M: Cancer Statistics, 2004. CA Cancer J Clin 2004; 54:8–29.

Koss LG: Diagnostic Cytology of the Urinary Tract. JB Lippincott, Philadelphia, 1995.

Murphy WM, Beckwith JB, Farrow GM: Tumors of the kidney, bladder, and related urinary structures in Atlas of Tumor Pathology, 3rd series, Fascicle 11. Armed Forces Institute of Pathology, Washington, DC, 1994, pp. 193–297.

Papanicolaou GN: Atlas of Exfoliative Cytology. Harvard University Press, Cambridge, MA, 1963.

Papanicolaou GN, and Marshall JF: Urine sediment smears as a diagnostic procedure in cancers of the urinary tract. Science 1945; 101:519.

Sarnaki CT, McCormack LJ, Kiser WS, et al: Urinary cytology and the clinical diagnosis of urinary tract malignancy: A clinicopathologic study of 1400 patients. J Urol 1977; 106:761.

Soloway MS, Briggman JV, Carpinito GA, Chodak GW, Church PA, Lamm DL, et al: Urine cytology and bladder cancer. J Urol 1996; 156:363–367.

1
Normal Morphology

Anatomic Considerations

The urinary tract can be divided into three regions: the kidney; the calyces, pelves and ureters (upper collecting system or upper tract); and the bladder and the urethra (lower collecting system or lower tract). From an exfoliative cytology standpoint, the kidneys are rarely of concern, for the tumors of the renal parenchyma are infrequently recovered in urinary specimens. Renal tumors are currently diagnosed pre-operatively either by their radiologic characteristics or by a Fine Needle Aspirate (FNA). Coverage of this topic is beyond the scope of this volume.

Normal Urothelial Histology and Cytology

The majority of the collecting system is lined by urothelium (transitional epithelium). Variable areas of the bladder and urethra may be lined by glandular epithelium (simple columnar), especially in the trigone and the dome of the bladder (the vestigial urachus); paraurethral glands, which provide lubrication for the urethra, might also be a source of glandular epithelium from that area. Cystitis cystica or glandularis, arising in Brunn's nests in the bladder mucosa, may shed groups of atypical glandular cells not to be confused with those cells of an adenocarcinoma of the bladder or prostate. In addition, the prostate and accessory sex glands are lined by columnar epithelium. Therefore, if glandular cells are seen within a urine sample, these sources should be considered.

The urothelium is a unique mucosa, specialized for the urinary tract for its ability to expand and contract, and as a barrier against the toxic urine. This stratified epithelium is morphologically intermediate between cuboidal and squamous, hence its old name, "transitional". When contracted, the bladder is lined by a layer 4–5 cells thick with the basal cells assuming a cuboidal shape; the intermediate cells, polygonal; and the surface cells round and large, and often binucleate. When the bladder is distended, the mucosa may be only 2–3 layers thick and the intermediate and surface cells may appear flattened.

The surface cells, the largest ones found in cytologic samples, have abundant cytoplasm, the luminal surface of which may appear thickened (Fig. 1.1). The nuclei of these superficial cells, often called umbrella cells, because of their position over more than one intermediate or basal cell (Fig. 1.2), may have prominent nucleoli, and may be multinucleated (Fig. 1.3).

The physiologic role of the urothelium is fascinating, and as unique as its cytologic appearance. The purpose of the urinary epithelium is to provide a barrier between the blood and the usually hypertonic toxic urine, which contains the majority of wastes from the body. The plasma membranes of the surface of umbrella cells are thicker than most other cell membranes. This rigid trilaminar membrane, the so-called "asymmetric unit membrane" is composed of a unique family of proteins, uroplakins. Interdigitating cell junctions permit great distension of the epithelium without damage to the integrity of the mucosal surface. The epithelium is connected to a basement membrane that appears invisible by light microscopy. The basal layer may be deeply indented by strands of underlying connective tissue which contain capillaries.

The histology of the other parts of the urinary tract, the ureters, pelves and calyces, and urethra, is essentially identical to the bladder, except that the size of the cells is smaller. Cross section of a contracted ureter reveals large mucosal folds that flatten if the ureter distends.

Columnar cells are infrequently present, but their identity is readily recognized as the cellular features are the same as any other benign columnar cell (Figs. 1.4, 1.5). Their origin may be in glandular remnants in the dome or trigone of the bladder. Urothelial cells on the surface of an hyperplasia may also appear to be columnar (Figs. 1.6, 1.7). Any atypia needs to be assessed in the context of accompanying inflammation, as from cystitis cystica/glandularis or suspicion of glandular neoplasia, based on history and cytologic features.

Squamous epithelium (Figs. 1.8, 1.9) can occur as a result of metaplasia or as a congenital area, especially within the trigone of women. The distal portion of the penile urethra is lined by squamous epithelium. In females, vaginal contamination during a voided urine collection (Fig. 1.10) can be a source of benign and neoplastic squamous and glandular epithelium (see Chapter 5).

8   1. Normal Morphology

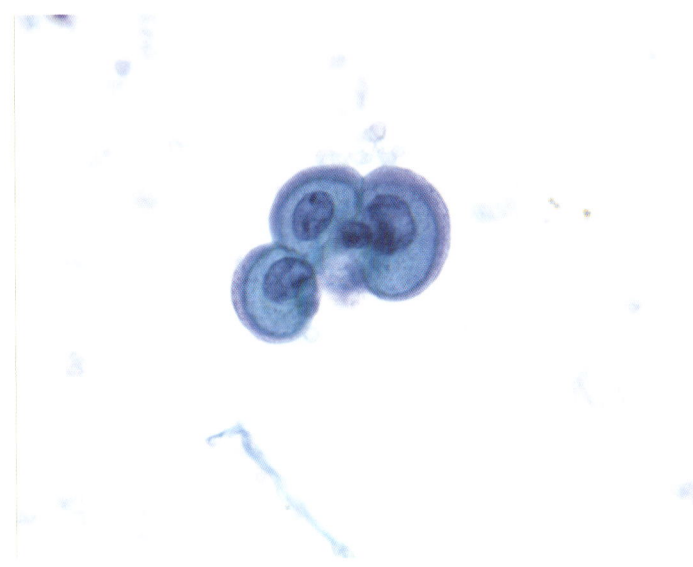

FIGURE 1.1. Normal Umbrella Cells—bladder washing: The thickened unilateral aspect of the cytoplasmic boundary is a manifestation of the asymmetric unit membrane whose purpose is to prevent toxic urine from entering the blood stream. In addition to the thickened asymmetric membrane, the frothy perinuclear cytoplasm is also characteristic of benign urothelial cells. Chromatin is fine and uniform in texture and distribution. (600x)

Normal Urothelial Histology and Cytology

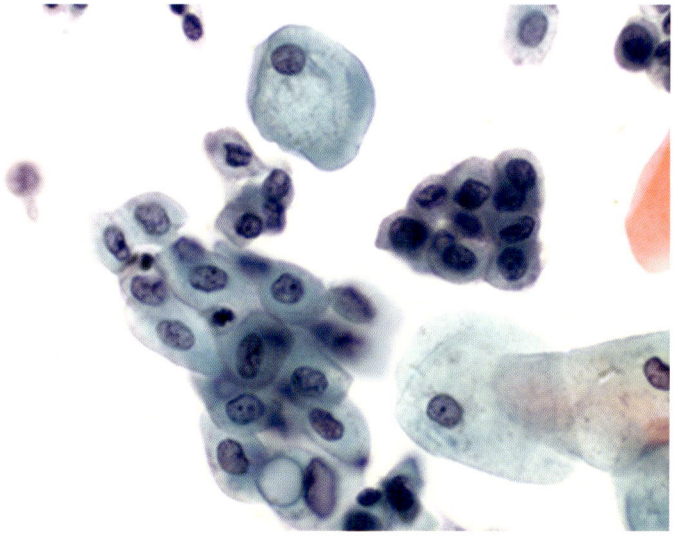

FIGURE 1.2. Benign Urothelial Cells—catheterized urine: Clusters of benign urothelial cells are admixed with squamous cells. Several acute inflammatory cells are seen in the background. The urothelial cells are seen in two main clusters, one cluster of which is smaller than the second. Cytoplasmic vacuolization and variability in nuclear size and shape is observed. Although the cytoplasm appears to be homogeneous, the nuclear cytoplasmic ratio is not increased. In catheterized specimens, these clusters represent benign or reactive urothelial cells. (600x)

10   1. Normal Morphology

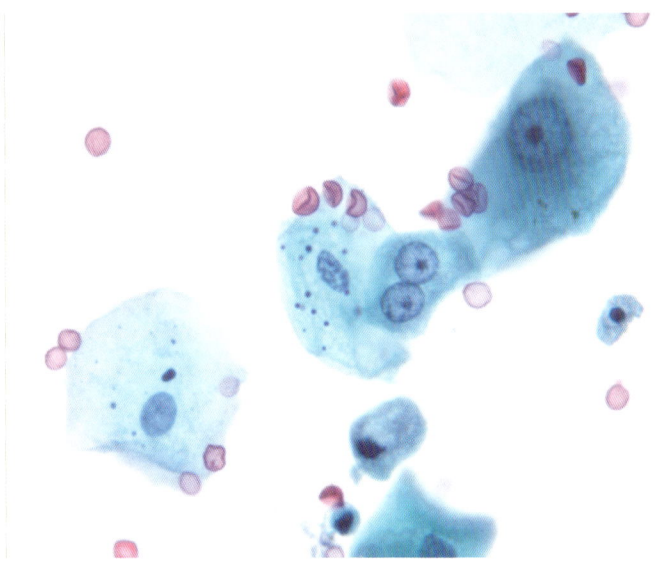

FIGURE 1.3. Normal Urothelial Cells—voided urine: Large round nuclei, frequently multiple, with prominent nucleoli are characteristic of normal umbrella (superficial) cells. Contrast these with the normal intermediate squamous cell in the lower left corner and in the center. (600x)

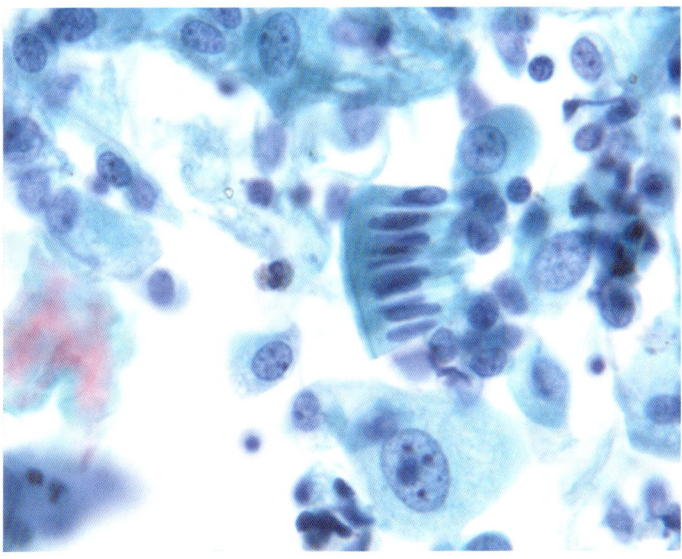

FIGURE 1.4. Glandular Cells—bladder washing: Columnar cells in a urinary specimen, if benign appearing, are of no clinical significance. They may arise in a focus of normal glandular epithelium in the bladder, but they may be mistaken for a glandular lesion. Cytomorphologic criteria should be applied as for any body site. (600x)

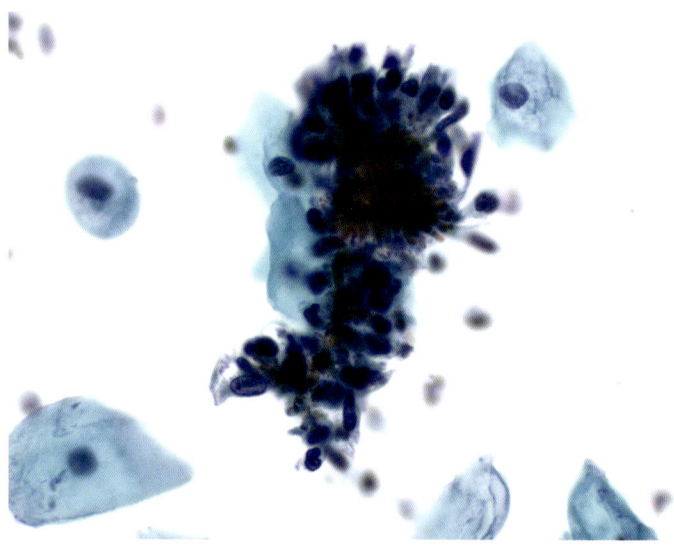

FIGURE 1.5. Glandular Cells—bladder washing: Elongated glandular cells surround degenerated debris. Follow-up showed endometriosis. (600x)

Normal Urothelial Histology and Cytology 13

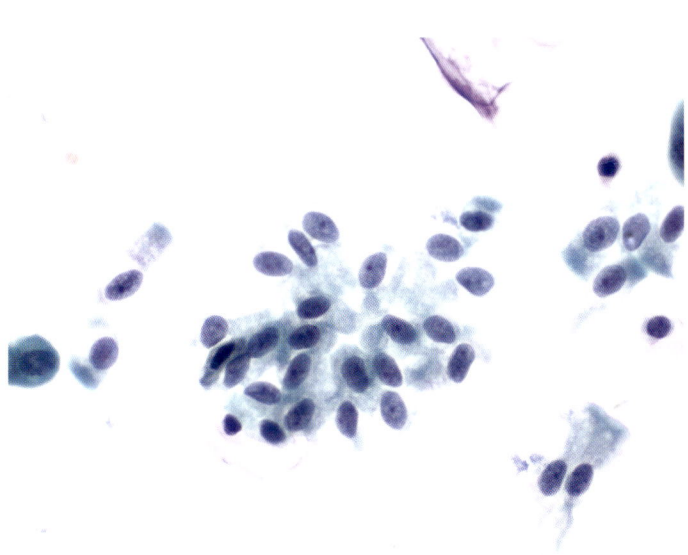

FIGURE 1.6. Benign Urothelial Cells—catheterized urine: In this catheterized urine, a loosely cohesive group of benign urothelial cells is present. These cells have an elongated glandular appearance. The cells have small dot-like nucleoli and abundant cytoplasm that is slightly frayed. (600x)

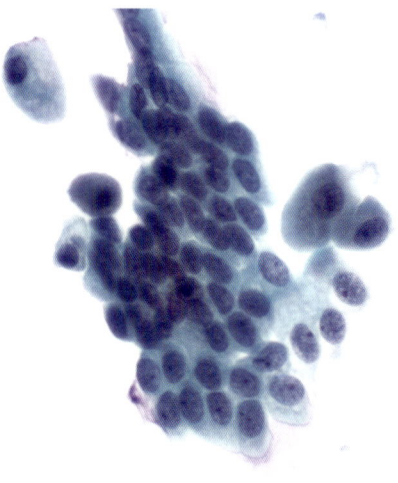

FIGURE 1.7. Benign Urothelial Cells—catheterized urine: A cluster of benign urothelial cells is admixed with scattered benign superficial cells. The cells have oval nuclei and frothy cytoplasm. The nuclear to cytoplasmic ratio is slightly increased although the nuclei are small. (600x)

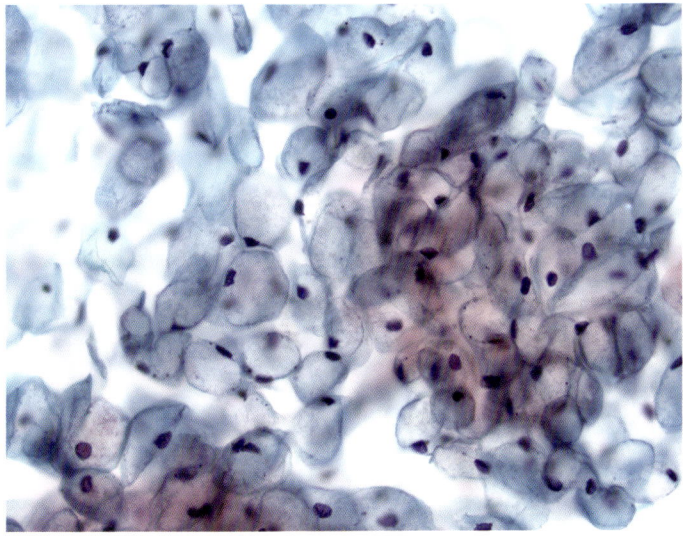

FIGURE 1.8. Benign Squamous Cells—voided urine: Numerous benign squamous cells are seen in this voided urine specimen from a 37 year old woman. The majority of these squamous cells are intermediate in appearance. These squamous cells may originate in the bladder or vagina. (600x)

16   1. Normal Morphology

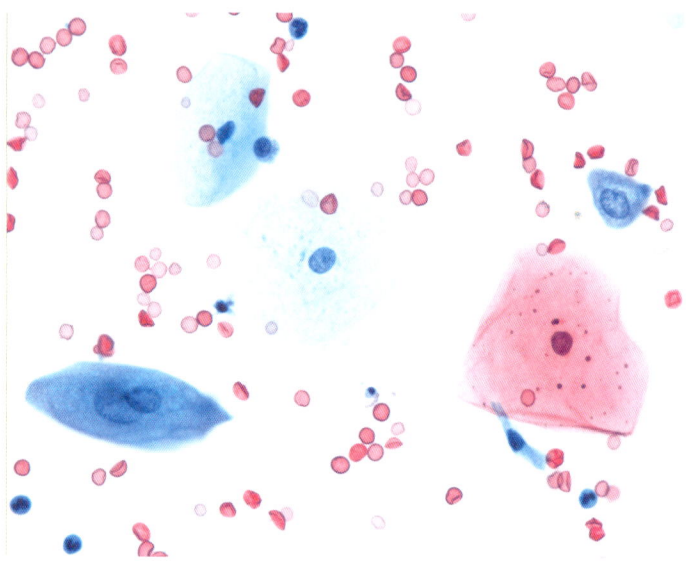

FIGURE 1.9. Normal Cells—voided urine: Normal urothelial cells are characterized by large round nuclei, often multiple, with prominent nucleoli and vesicular cytoplasm. In this photograph, several squamous cells are present and are characteristically without nucleoli. (400x)

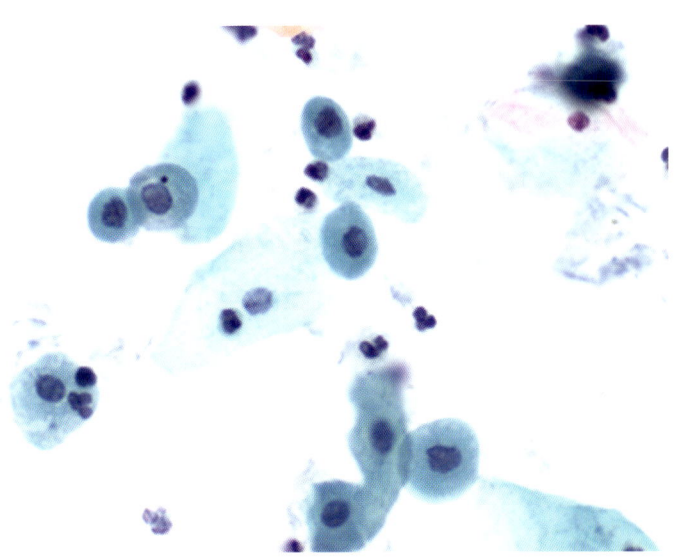

FIGURE 1.10. Vaginal Contaminant—voided urine: Acute inflammation and benign squamous cells admixed with bacteria are seen in the background. Benign urothelial cells also are present. In some voided urines, vaginal contaminant may obscure the benign urothelial cells. (600x)

Suggested Reading

Dabbs DJ: Cytology of pyelitis glandularis cystica. Acta Cytol 1992; 36:943–945.

Epstein JI, Amin MB, Reuter VR, Mostofi FK, and the Bladder Consensus Conference Committee: The World Health Organization/International Society of Urological Pathology consensus classification of urothelial (transitional cell) neoplasms of the urinary bladder. Am J of Surg Path 1998; 22:1435–1448.

Koss LG: Diagnostic Cytology of the Urinary Tract. JB Lippincott, Philadelphia, 1995.

2
Diagnostic Categories

Formatting the Report

Communication with the clinician is incredibly important, especially for lesions of the upper tract and borderline changes. Unfortunately, there has yet to be a concensus conference on terminology for urothelial cytology. Therefore, we propose the following categories be adopted (Table 1).

No cytologic atypia
Benign cellular changes
Atypia indeterminate for neoplasia
Low grade neoplasia
High grade neoplasia
Unsatisfactory

Needless to say, modifiers to neoplastic categories, such as "suspicious for" or "suggestive of" are the prerogatives of the pathologist, and expected/accepted by our clinical colleagues. Repeat cytologic sampling or further diagnostic studies should ensue in these cases.

Criteria for unsatisfactory specimens are not defined. Voided urines are usually less cellular than bladder washings, and will vary depending upon the processing method routinely utilized. At least 25cc of freshly collected urine should be recommended for adequate cell retrieval in voided urine. The prudent pathologist will develop an eye for the usual cellularity for both voided and washed samples in his/her laboratory. When a sample has obscuring

TABLE 1. Comparative Features of Major Categories of Urothelial Conditions

	Normal	Reactive	Atypical	Low Grade	High Grade
Cellularity	Single	Single	Groups	Fragments	Single/groups
Cytoplasm	Textured, pale	Bubbley	Variable	Opaque	Variable
Nucleus-size	Small	Enlarged	Variable	Larger	Variable, large
Nucleus-shape	Round	Round	Irregular	Oval	Very irregular
Nucleoli	Tiny	Obvious	Variable	Absent	Often large
Chromatin	Pale, uniform	Coarse, uniform	Variable	Uniform, darker	Irregular, dark
N/C	Low	Increased	Variable	Increased	High
Background	Clean	Inflamed	Clean or inflamed	Clean or bloody	Variable

lubricant in a washing (Fig. 2.1), or is very hypo-cellular in either type of sample, a diagnosis of "Unsatisfactory" is advised, unless there is any hint of significant atypia. Then the diagnosis must express the morphologic changes and mention the scant cellularity or obscuring factors as a quality indicator.

Morphologic Differences Dependent on Method of Sample Collection

While the nuclear criteria may not provide evidence of neoplasia, the growth pattern is oftentimes a significant clue to the ongoing process. Sampling method will alter the composition of the specimen, and is important to know before rendering an interpretation (Table 2).

In spontaneously voided urine, a sufficient sample for diagnosis may not be obtained. Large pseudopapillary cellular groups should cause concern in a voided specimen, particularly if the clinical history is unknown. The differential diagnosis includes instrumentation artifact, resulting in large groups of urothelial cells (Fig. 2.2–2.7). Catheterization will avoid vaginal contamination in a woman and establish the source of blood, i.e., bladder vs. uterus. An irrigation specimen obtained during cystoscopy is the best source of adequate epithelium to appreciate crowding produced by increased

TABLE 2. Cytologic Differences Depending on Collection Techniques

	Voided	Catheterized	Washing	Loop
Cellularity	Low	Higher	Highest	Usually high
Preservation	Poor-medium	Better	Good	Degenerated
Architecture	Single cells	Fragments	Groups and fragments	Groups and single
Cell types	Umbrella	Umbrella, basal	Umbrella, basal	Enteric, umbrella
Advantages	Non-invasive	Better specimen	Best specimen	None
Disadvantages	Degeneration, scant, vaginal contamination	Instrumentation artifact, infection	Invasive, antibiotic prophylaxis	Degeneration

NC ratios, minimal increase in nuclear size, chromatin quality and perhaps a mildly disordered arrangement of cells. Comparison with normal urothelium produced by irrigation in the same sample will prevent over-calling these usually cellular samples (Figs. 2.8–2.10). Needless to say, clinicians are responsible for noting on the requisiton the method of collection. If lubricant is present (Fig. 2.11) a voided sample is not a possibility; cell groups should be attributed to mechanical disruption rather than to neoplasia, unless the individual cell features and architecture within the fragments persuade otherwise.

Benign Cellular Changes—Normal/Reactive

Normal urothelial cells have bland nuclear chromatin, uniformly round nuclei, inconspicuous nucleoli, and frothy cytoplasm. Reactive/inflammatory changes in urothelial cells are similar to those of all epithelial cells, i.e., accentuated nucleoli, slightly coarsened chromatin, round nuclei and a variably increased nuclear-cytoplasmic (NC) ratio (Figs. 2.12–2.14, 2.16–2.19). In contrast, cells from low grade urothelial carcinoma have oval nuclei, indiscernible nucleoli, and high NC ratios (Figs. 3.7–3.19)

Most infectious agents are not obvious in voided urine or washings, but occasionally trichomonads, evidence of polyoma virus (decoy cells) (Figs. 2.20, 2.21), Herpes simplex virus

(Figs. 2.22, 2.23), cytomegalovirus (CMV) (Fig. 2.24) or human papillomavirus (koilocytes) is seen (Figs. 2.25). Schistoma ova are found rarely in our practice, but should be sought when extensive squamous metaplasia is seen.

Renal tubular epithelial cells are usually so degenerated by the time they reach the bladder that they resemble histiocytes (Fig. 2.26). They are usually few in number, unless there is intrinsic renal disease affecting the tubules. Cellular casts preserve the cytomorphology of these cells (Fig. 2.27), and are important to report.

Benign Non-epithelial Elements

Cytology reports should include not only cellular elements, but also other features that have clinical significance. These include casts, crystals, inclusions (Figs. 2.28–2.32), and ejaculate which may include seminal vesicle cells, not to be mistaken for neoplastic cells.

Atypical Urothelial Cells Indeterminate for Neoplasia

Unfortuntely, as in every other body site, cytologic samples from the urinary tract are not always readily placed into distinct categories. An atypical interpretation is appropriate when morphologic changes exceed those described as benign cellular changes, but lack clear signs of neoplasia (Figs. 2.7, 2.15, 2.33). This is generally encountered when dealing with a sample from a patient with a low grade lesion, especially those called "low malignant potential" (LMP), or in the presence of severe inflammation, calculus disease, or following chemotherapy. Emerging ancillary tests, beyond the scope of this volume, will potentially bring clarity to these frustrating lesions.

Note that "dysplasia" is not included as a diagnostic choice. In the authors' experience, cytologic samples rarely contain cells from a dysplasia unless they have been mechanically dislodged. If they are present, they should be placed in a low or high grade category depending upon individual cell morphology.

Benign Cellular Changes 23

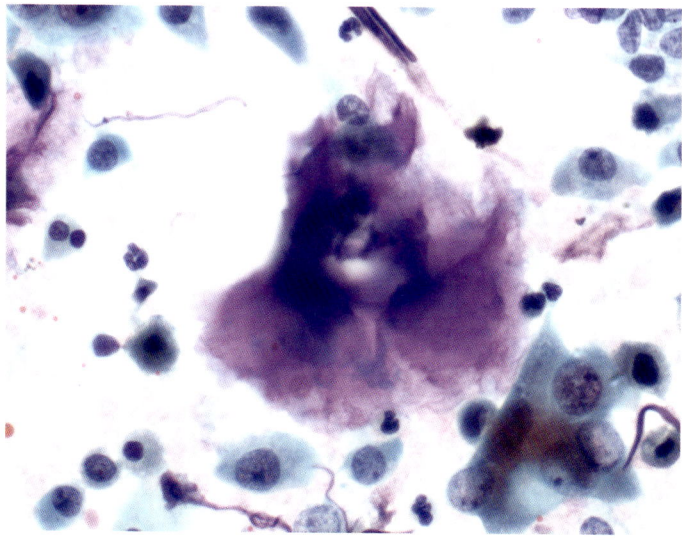

FIGURE 2.1. Benign Urothelial Cells—bladder washing: The purple fragment is lubricant. Admixed are acute inflammatory cells as well as reactive urothelial cells. Lubricant may be seen in bladder washing and catheterized specimens. (600x)

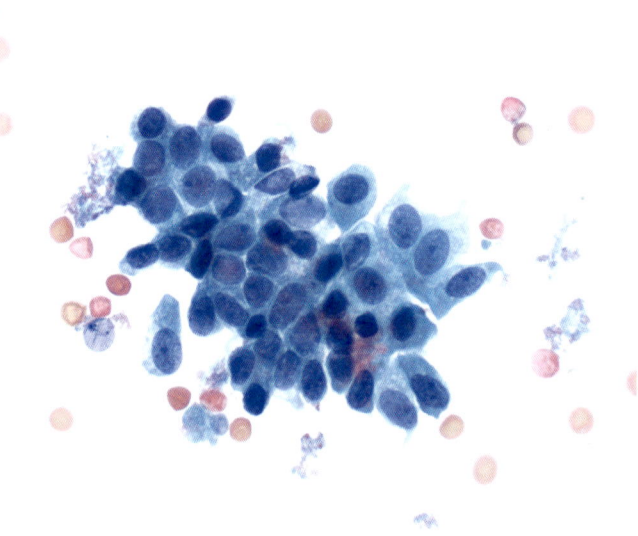

FIGURE 2.2. Benign Urothelial Cells—catheterized urine: Degeneration may be seen in catheterized urine specimens. In this case, degenerated nuclei are admixed with smaller, hyperchromatic benign urothelial cells. (600x)

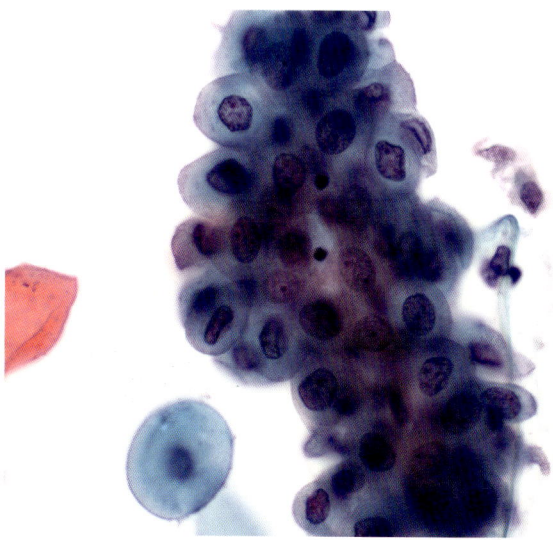

FIGURE 2.3. Benign Urothelial Cells—catheterized urine: A cluster of benign urothelial cells is admixed with a few squamous cells. The urothelial cells exhibit a moderately increased nuclear to cytoplasmic ratio although the nuclei are relatively uniform to slightly irregular in contour. The cells contain a variable chromatin pattern and the cytoplasm is homogeneous (absence of vacuoles). Clusters of benign urothelial cells in catheterized urine specimens should not be mistaken for low or high grade urothelial carcinoma. (600x)

FIGURE 2.4. Benign Urothelial Cells—catheterized urine: In this catheterized urine, a large group of benign urothelial cells is present at a low power. At this power, one may be concerned for a low grade urothelial carcinoma. However, such large clusters are often seen in catheterized urine specimens and should not evoke a low grade carcinoma diagnosis. (200x)

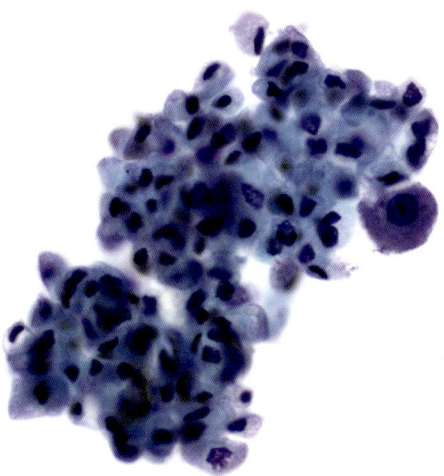

FIGURE 2.5. Reactive Urothelial Cells—catheterized urine: A large cluster of degenerated, benign, reactive urothelial cells is seen. These cells exhibit low nuclear to cytoplasmic ratios although the nuclei are irregular in contour. The nuclear to cytoplasmic ratio is not increased. Several of the cells show marked hyperchromasia, although degeneration explains this phenomenon. (600x)

28   2. Diagnostic Categories

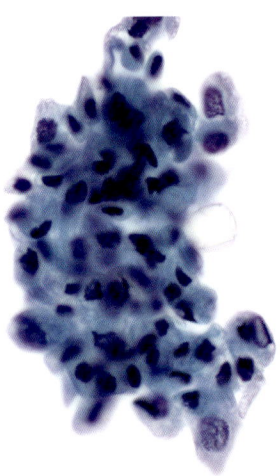

FIGURE 2.6. Reactive Urothelial Cells—catheterized urine: A cluster of benign, degenerated urothelial cells is seen adjacent to a crystal. The more preserved urothelial cells contain enlarged nuclei that are not hyperchromatic and may be seen at the edges of the large cluster. For the most part, the nuclei are small and hyperchromatic. (600x)

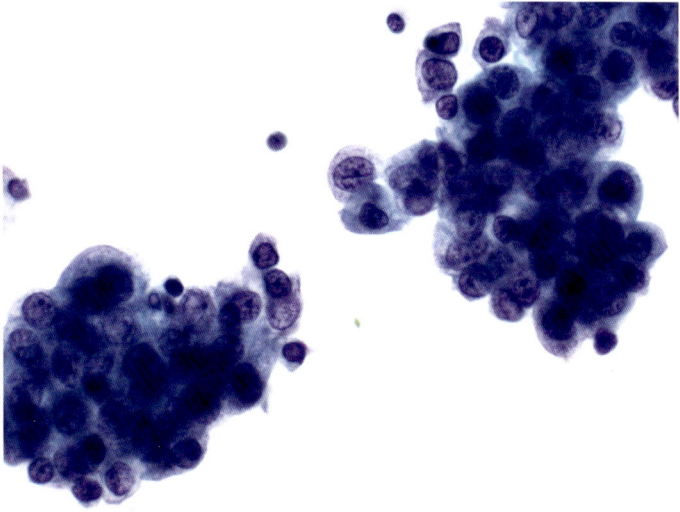

FIGURE 2.7. Atypical Urothelial Cells—catheterized urine: Two large clusters of atypical urothelial cells are seen. The cells exhibit an increased nuclear to cytoplasmic ratio although the nuclei are not markedly hyperchromatic. The cytoplasm is granular and there is an absence of cytoplasmic homogeneity. Nuclear overlap may be seen in catheterized specimens and in this case, the nuclei vary in size, although for the most part are round in shape. (600x)

30 2. Diagnostic Categories

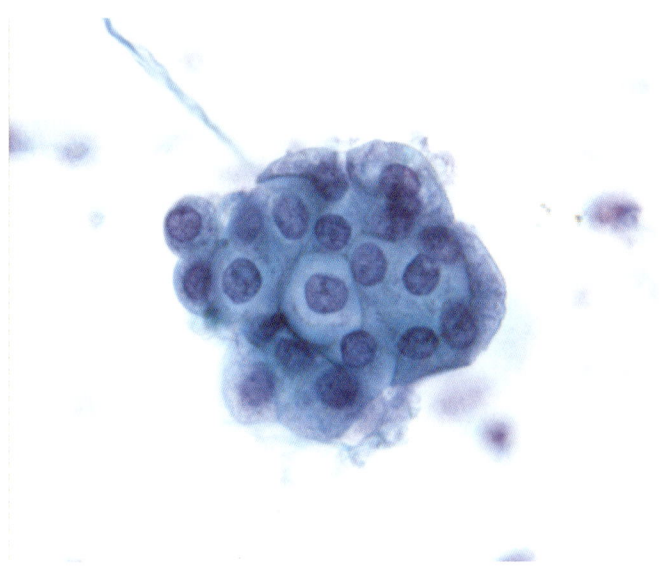

FIGURE 2.8. Normal Umbrella Cells—bladder washing: Instrumentation will usually produce tissue fragments. The distinct cellular outlines, frothy cytoplasm and relatively round, uniform nuclei testify to their benign nature. (600x)

Benign Cellular Changes 31

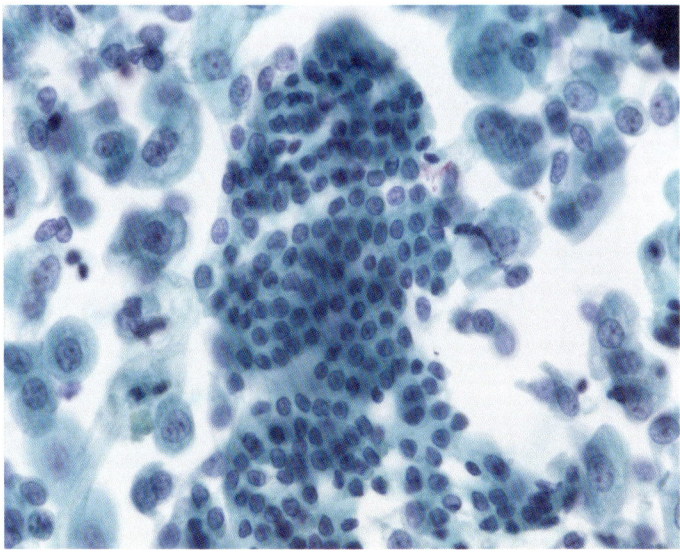

FIGURE 2.9. Normal Cells: Bladder washing can produce sheets of normal urothelial cells as well as single umbrella cells. This illustration displays the smaller nuclei of the basal cells in comparison with the larger nuclei of umbrella cells surrounding the tissue fragment. Note that the boundaries of this tissue fragment are not smooth (compare with low grade papillary lesion in Figure 3.7). (400x)

32   2. Diagnostic Categories

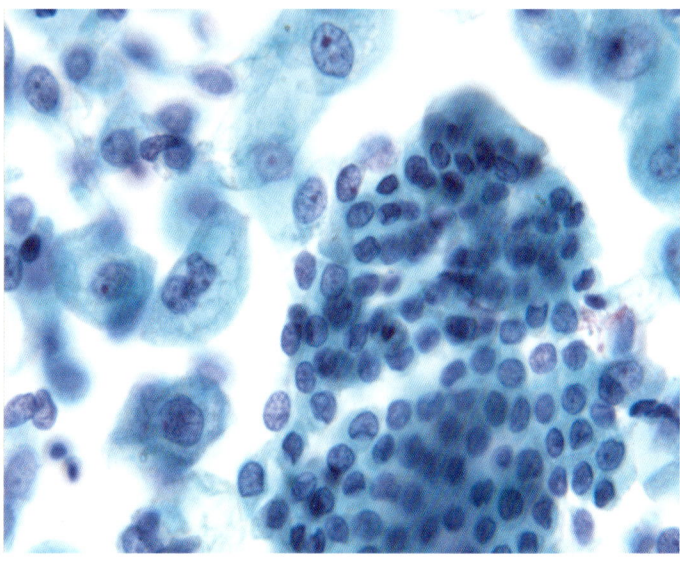

FIGURE 2.10. Normal Urothelial Cells—bladder washing: A fragment of basal urothelial cells is surrounded by single umbrella cells. Note the smaller nuclei of the basal cells when compared with the umbrella cells which also feature prominent nucleoli. (600x)

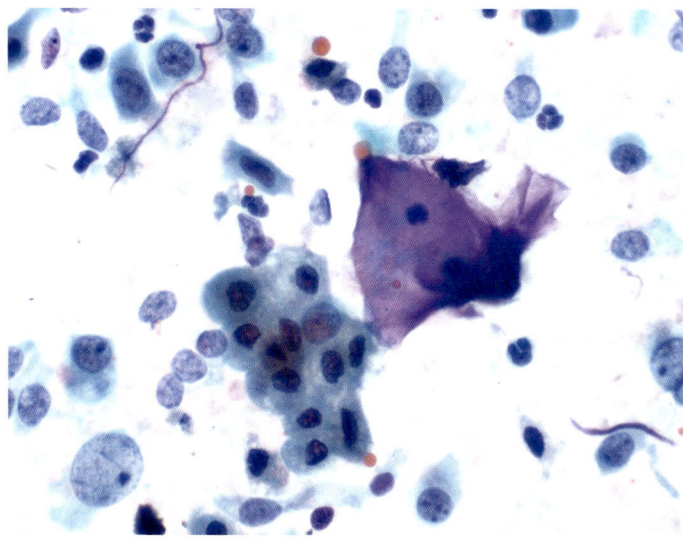

FIGURE 2.11. Lubricant—bladder washing: A fragment of lubricant is admixed with benign urothelial cells. (600x)

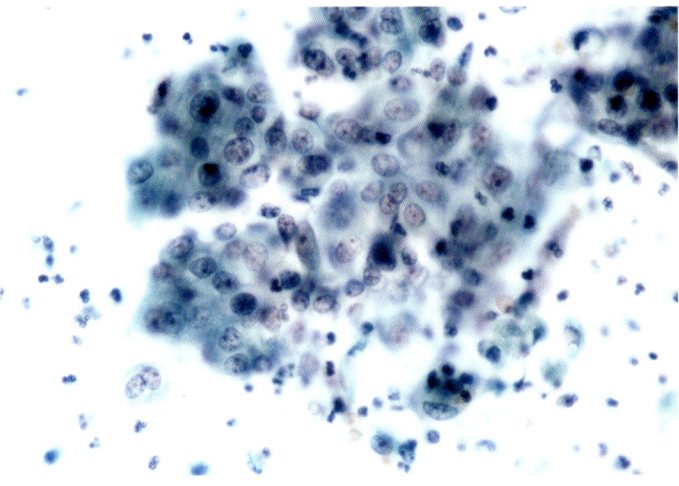

FIGURE 2.12. Reactive Urothelial Cells—bladder washing: Sheets of epithelial cells may be misinterpreted as neoplastic. Careful examination of nuclear criteria, such as pale chromatin, prominent nucleoli, low NC ratios, and a background of acute inflammation, contributes to the interpretation of reactive/inflammatory cellular changes. (200x)

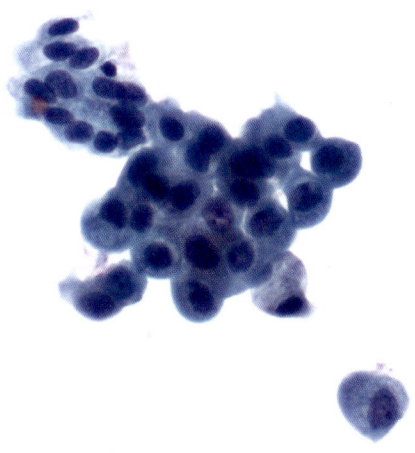

FIGURE 2.13. Reactive Urothelial Cells—bladder washing: These urothelial cells show slightly increased nuclear to cytoplasmic ratios and variably sized nuclei. The cytoplasm is homogeneous and only mildly atypical. (600x)

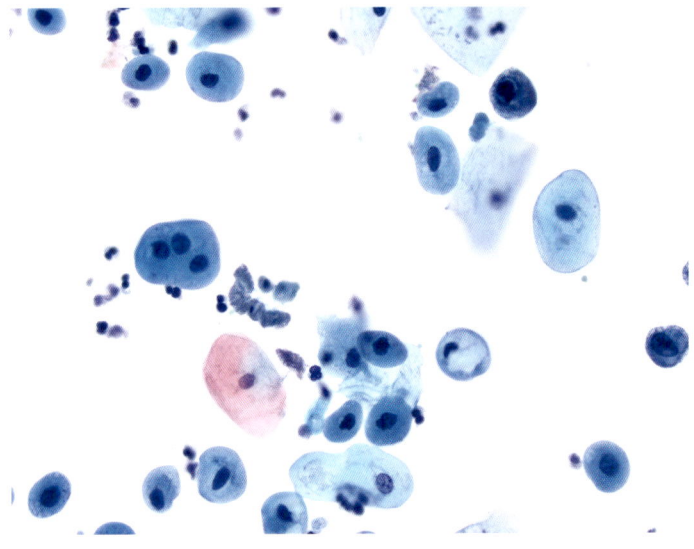

Figure 2.14. Reactive Urothelial Cells—bladder washing: Numerous neutrophils, benign squamous cells and reactive urothelial cells are present. Several of the cells show degeneration and nuclear hyperchromasia. The nuclear to cytoplasmic ratio of the cells is not significantly increased. (600x)

Benign Cellular Changes 37

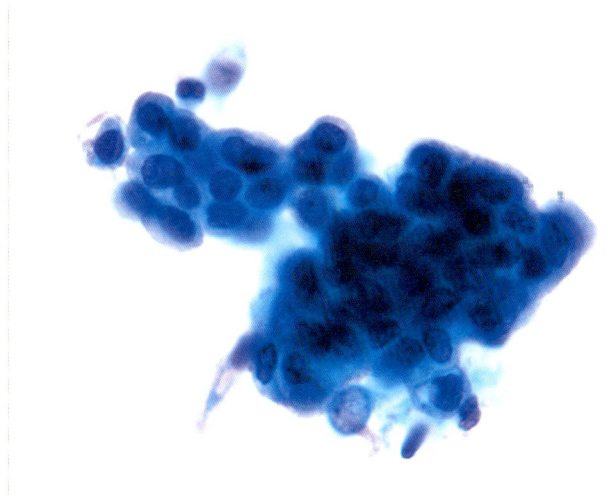

FIGURE 2.15. Atypical Urothelial Cells Indeterminate for Neoplasia—renal pelvic brushing: This fragment of urothelial cells was originally considered atypical without all the features of a low grade neoplasm. Note the high NC ratios, variable nuclear shapes, and hyperchromasia. Other areas of the same sample had more atypical cells reflecting the lesion, a Papillary Urothelial Neoplasm of Low Malignant Potential. See Figure 3.2. (600x)

38   2. Diagnostic Categories

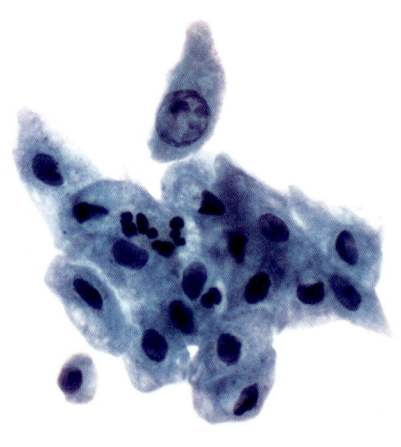

FIGURE 2.16. Reactive Urothelial Cells—bladder washing: A cluster of reactive urothelial cells is seen. The cells are admixed with acute inflammatory cells and show either marked nuclear hyperchromasia and degeneration or a prominent nucleolus. (600x)

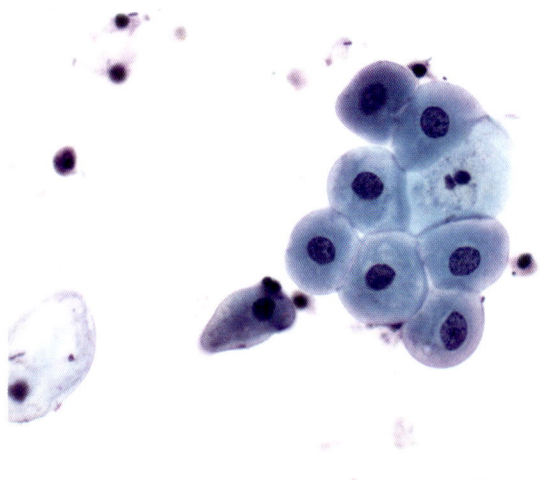

FIGURE 2.17. Reactive Urothelial Cells—catheterized urine: These superficial reactive urothelial cells show homogeneous cytoplasm and mildly hyperchromatic nuclei. Note the low nuclear to cytoplasmic ratio, acute inflammation and bacteria in the background. (600x)

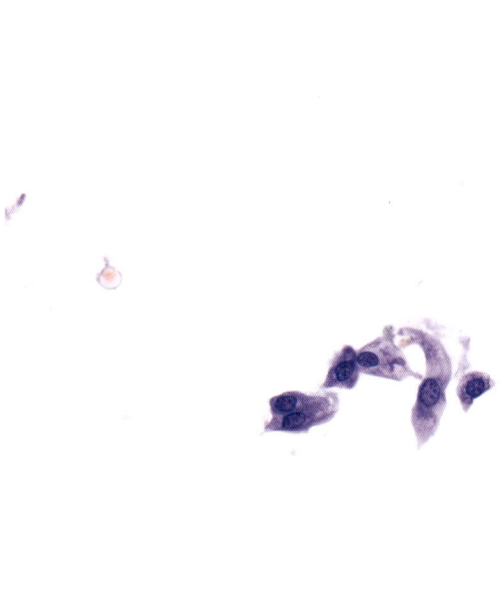

FIGURE 2.18. Reactive Urothelial Cells—bladder washing: Degenerated reactive urothelial cells are seen. These cells exhibit nuclear membrane irregularities and nuclear hyperchromasia. These cells also have a large amount of cytoplasm, indicative of their benign nature. (600x)

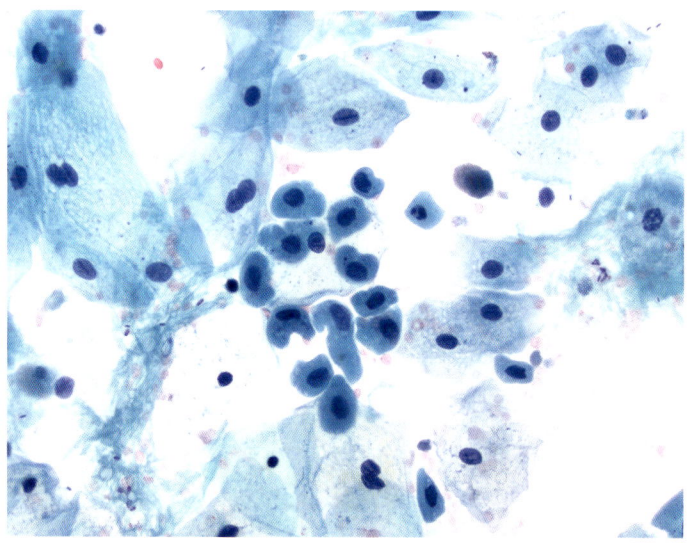

FIGURE 2.19. Reactive Urothelial Cells—bladder washing: Degenerated slightly atypical urothelial cells are seen. The cells exhibit only mildly increased nuclear to cytoplasmic ratios and many of the cells contain abundant cytoplasm. Note that the nuclear size is smaller than the size of intermediate squamous cells. (600x)

42   2. Diagnostic Categories

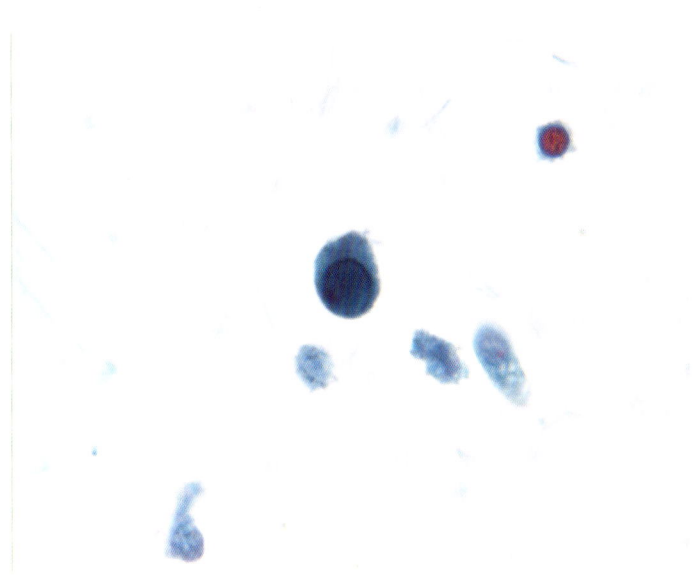

FIGURE 2.20. Polyoma Virus—voided urine: If this is a rare cell in the specimen, then one can presume a viral infection. However, nuclear changes could be degeration in a cell from a high grade carcinoma and warrant careful follow-up. (600x)

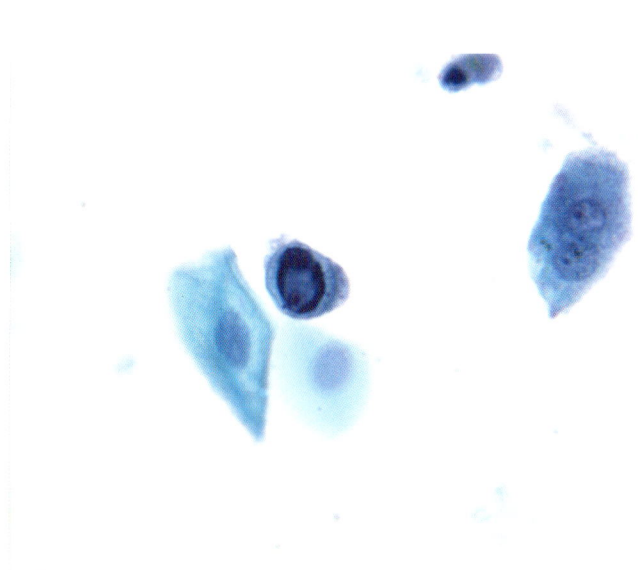

FIGURE 2.21. Polyoma Virus—voided urine: An infected cell displays overall cell enlargement, high NC ratio, and ground glass nucleus with marginated chromatin. Compare the infected cell with the adjacent benign urothelial cell. (600x).

2. Diagnostic Categories

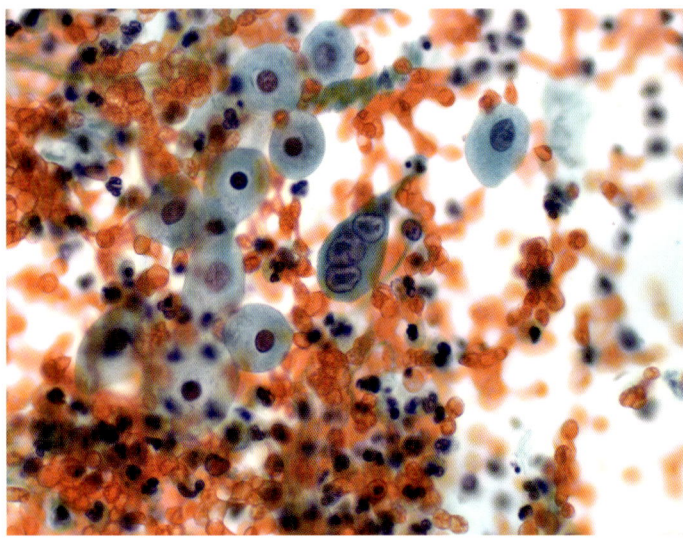

FIGURE 2.22. Herpes Simplex Infection—voided urine: A cell with herpetic viral inclusions is seen in the center field admixed with blood, benign urothelial cells and acute inflammation. The herpetic cell exhibits a multilobated nucleus and a relatively low nuclear to cytoplasmic ratio. The cytoplasm appears homogeneous. (600x)

Benign Cellular Changes 45

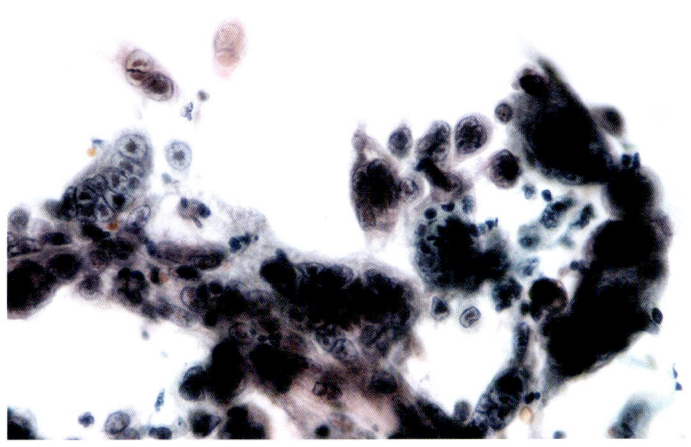

FIGURE 2.23. Herpes Simplex Infection—urethral brushing: Intranuclear inclusions, multinucleation and nuclear molding typify Herpes infection anywhere in the body. This patient had AIDS, and died of systemic Herpes infection. (400x)

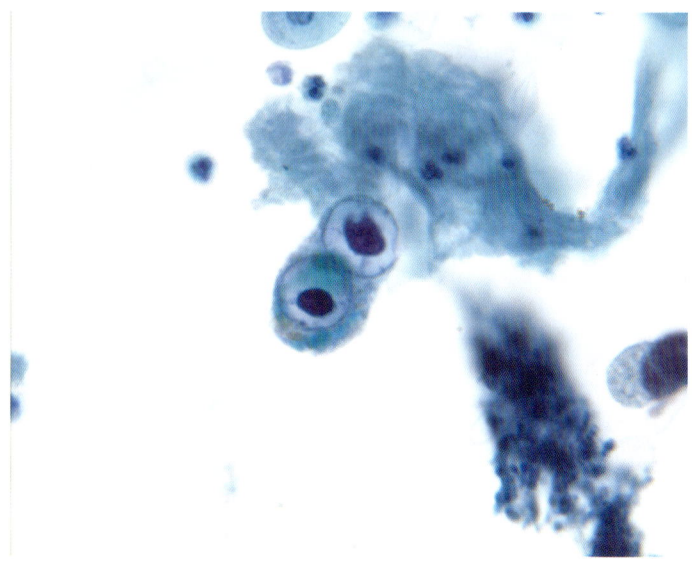

FIGURE 2.24. Cytomegalovirus Infected Urothelial Cells—voided urine: In urines, viral cytopathic effect is characteristically similar to CMV infections in other body sites. Compare these enlarged nuclei with distinct intranuclear inclusions and perinuclear clearing with the nuclear changes produced by polyoma virus infection. They are distinctly and diagnostically different. (600x)

Benign Cellular Changes 47

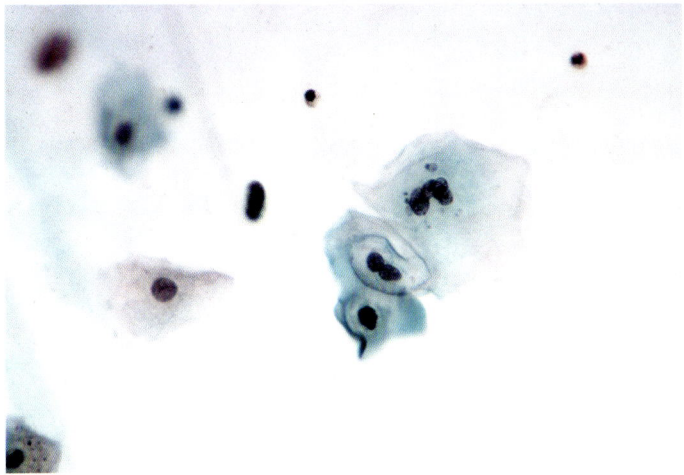

FIGURE 2.25. Human Papillomavirus Infection—bladder washing: Koilocytes, the hallmark of HPV infection, can be found rarely in urologic specimens. They may originate from genital contamination in voided urines obtained from female patients. This patient was male, the specimen was obtained by bladder washing, and the lesion was biopsy proven to be a bladder condyloma. (400x)

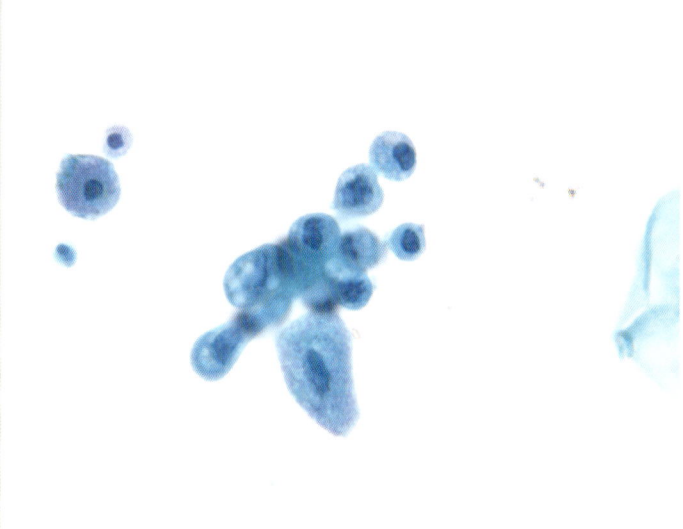

FIGURE 2.26. Renal Tubular Epithelial Cells—voided urine: As their name implies, these cells derive from the lining cells of the renal tubules. They mimic macrophages because of their degenerated, often eccentric, nucleus and foamy cytoplasm. The larger cell in the bottom of the figure is a normal umbrella cell. (600x)

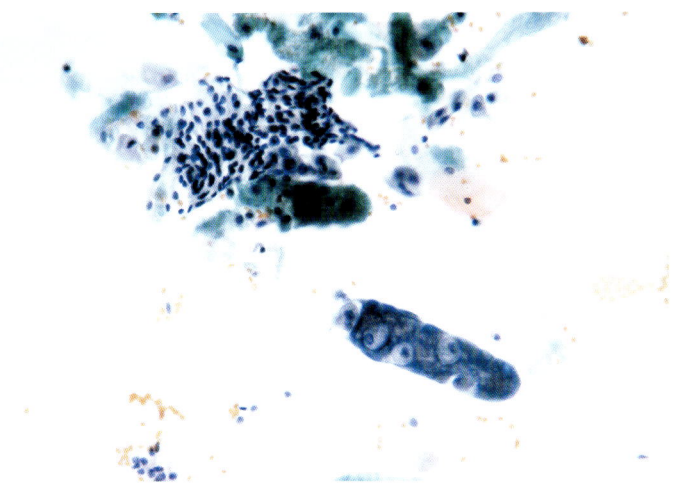

FIGURE 2.27. Tubular Cast—voided urine: Renal tubular epithelial cells have usually degenerated by the time they are recovered in voided urine. This cast has preserved the morphology without any degeneration, much like a fossil preserves features of long dead creatures. (200x)

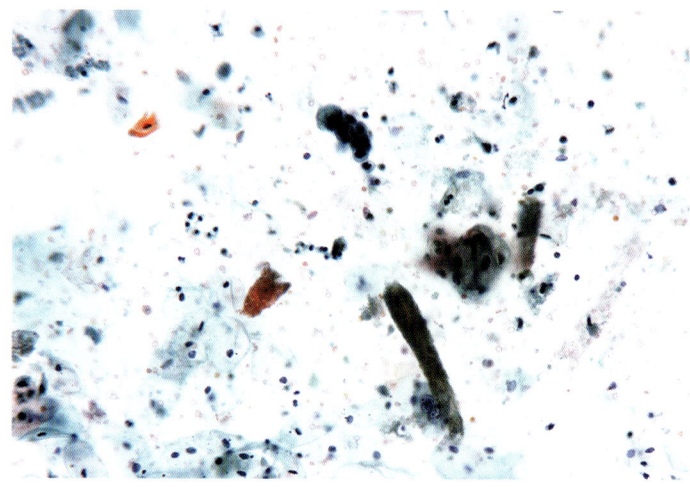

FIGURE 2.28. Assorted Casts—voided urine: Types of casts can be important clinical information and should be mentioned in addition to any epithelial atypia. (200x)

Benign Non-epithelial Elements   51

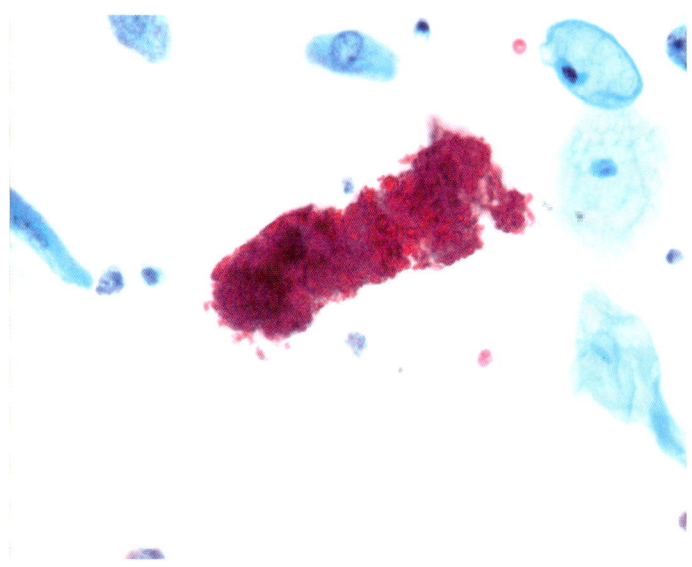

Figure 2.29. Red Cell Casts—voided urine: Fragmented red blood cells are arranged in a cylinder with relatively parallel sides. (400x)

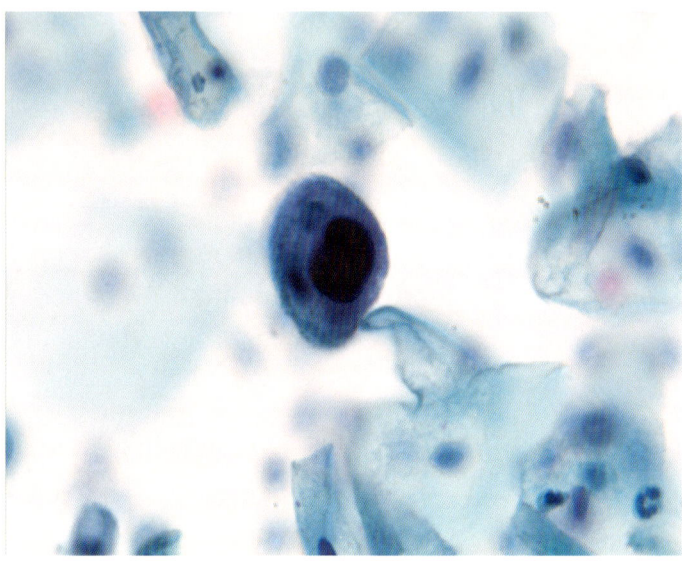

FIGURE 2.30. Non-viral Inclusions—voided urine: Red opaque inclusions in large degenerated spheres are not to be confused with virus infected cells. The exact origin of these inclusions is not known. They do not correlate with any disease process. They are a frequent finding in voided urines, especially in the presense of inflammation and in older patients. (600x)

Benign Non-epithelial Elements 53

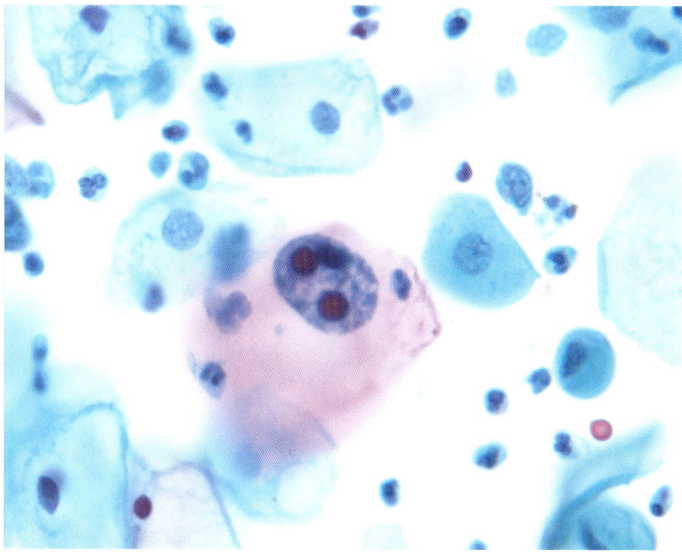

FIGURE 2.31. Non-viral Inclusions—voided urine: Red inclusions within degenerated cells are frequently seen in voided urines and are of no apparent clinical significance. They usually accompany acute inflammation. (600x)

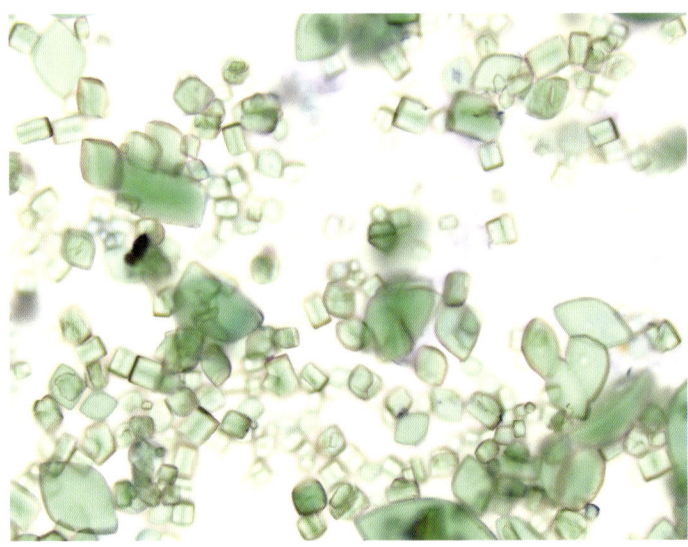

FIGURE 2.32. Benign Crystals—bladder washing: Numerous crystals are seen in this bladder washing specimen. The crystals range in size and shape and few benign urothelial cells are observed. (600x)

Atypical Urothelial Cells Indeterminate for Neoplasia

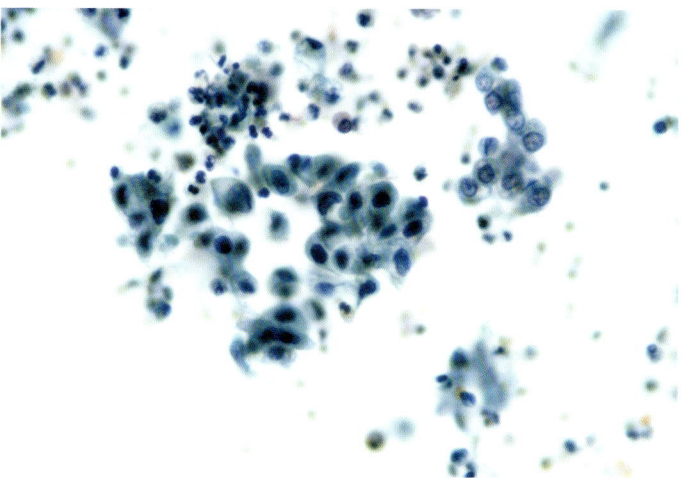

FIGURE 2.33. Atypical Cells, Short of Neoplastic—bladder washing: When cytologic criteria fall between reactive and neoplastic, an indeterminate category is prudent. Clinical management usually includes repeat voided urines, followed by bladder washing and biopsy if atypical cells persist. (400x)

Suggested Reading

Boon ME, van Keep JM, and Kok LP: Polyomavirus infection versus high grade bladder carcinoma. Acta Cytol 1989; 33:887–893.

Layfield LJ, Elsheikh TM, Fili A, Nayar R, Shidham V. Review of the state of the art and recommendations of the Papanicolaou Society of Cytopathology for urinary cytology procedures and reporting. Diagn Cytopathol 2004;30:24–30.

Roussel F, Picquenot J-M, and Rousseau O: Identification of human papillomavirus antigen in a bladder tumor. Acta Cytol 1991; 35:273–276.

Santos RL, Manfrinatto JA, Cia EM, Carvalho RB, Quadros KR, Alves-Filho G, Mazzali M. Urine cytology as a screening method for polyoma virus active infection. Transplant Proc. 2004;36:899–901.

3
Grading Urothelial Neoplasms (Transitional Cell Carcinoma, TCC)

Terminology

Historic

Historically, terminology describing urinary tract lesions has been almost as confusing as lymphoma categories. A popular histologic grading system divides the neoplasms into three groups: Grade I (low), Grade II (medium), and Grade III (high). In those systems that add a fourth grade, equivalence may be accomplished by placing papillomas in the Grade I category, the low grade lesions in Grade II, etc. Including papillomas with Grade I lesions may be justified by the evidence that these benign appearing papillomas may progress to higher grade carcinomas, or at least identify the patient as at risk for subsequent development of a high grade lesion. From a patient management standpoint, all papillary lesions of the urinary bladder can be considered cancerous. However, the current general opinion, that the most treacherous lesions are the high grade sessile (flat) lesions, capable of quickly invading, makes the low grade papillary lesions less noteworthy than previously considered. Therefore, cytopathologists may prefer to divide the neoplasms of the urothelium simply into low and high grade.

TABLE 3. The WHO/ISUP Consensus Classification

Normal
    May include cases formerly diagnosed as "mild dysplasia"
Hyperplasia
    Flat hyperplasia
    Papillary hyperplasia
Flat lesions with atypia
    Reactive (inflammatory) atypia
    Atypia of unknown significance
    Dysplasia (low grade intraurothelial neoplasia)
    Carcinoma in situ (high grade intraurothelial neoplasia)
Papillary neoplasms
    Papilloma—Inverted papilloma
    Papillary neoplasm of low malignant potential (PUNLMP)
    Papillary carcinoma, low grade
    Papillary carcinoma, high grade
Invasive neoplasms
    Lamina propria invasion
    Muscularis propria (detrusor muscle) invasion

Terminology used in this Handbook

The newest terminology considers the natural history of urothelial neoplasia and the relationship to premalignant and preinvasive lesions. In 1998, members of the International Society of Urologic Pathologists (ISUP) met to discuss bladder terminology and make recommendations to the World Health Organization (WHO) Committee on urothelial tumors. The resulting Consensus Classification of Urothelial (Transitional Cell) Neoplasms of the Urinary Bladder is outlined on Table 3. Comparison with previous popular terminologies is tabulated on Table 4.

Conveniently, the new classification closely "fits" the way in which most cytopathologists categorize urinary cytologic samples (Table 5). Since the morphologic changes in the lowest grade lesions are essentially identical to normal urothelium, the sensitivity of cytology for the accurate diagnosis of these tumors is low. Hyperplasia is included in the categories of the WHO/ISUP classification, but is rarely recognized in a cytologic specimen (Fig. 3.1). However, the risk that a low grade lesion may progress to invasive carcinoma is minimal, reducing the negative consequences of a false negative. High grade lesions fortunately are easily recognized and reliably

TABLE 4. Histologic Grading Systems for Urothelial Carcinoma and Cytologic Equivalents

	Cytologic Equivalent	1998 WHO/ISUP	Murphy	1973 WHO
Flat lesions	Reactive/inflammatory changes	Reactive Atypia or Atypia of unknown significance	None	None
	Atypia indeterminate for neoplasia	Dysplasia	None	None
	High grade urothelial carcinoma	Carcinoma in Situ	None	None
Papillary lesions	Normal cells, clusters in voided urine	Papilloma	Papilloma	Papilloma
	Normal or atypical cells	Low Malignant Potential (LMP)	Low grade	Grade 1
	Atypical cells/low grade carcinoma	Low grade	High grade	Grade 2
	High grade urothelial carcinoma	High grade	High grade	Grade 3

diagnosed so that immediate histologic confirmation and treatment can proceed.

Low Grade Urothelial Tumors (Grade I, Papilloma, Papillary Urothelial Neoplasm of Low Malignant Potential)

Diagnosis	Cytologic Criteria
Papillary Neoplasm Of Low Malignant Potential (LMP) (Grade I)	chromatin coarseness loss of "honeycomb" nuclear shape elongated nuclear enlargement nucleoli indistinct umbrella cells retained

According to most authors, the cytologic diagnosis of low grade urothelial lesions is made with difficulty. One of the obvious reasons is that these lesions do not shed as readily as the higher grade lesions, and therefore the amount of diagnosable material in a given sample is small. Another reason is that the DNA content of these tumors is at or near diploid, and so the nuclear chromatin of these cells is essentially identical to that of the normal mucosa. The low grade lesions exhibit a spectrum of features from changes identical to benign urothelium (as in papilloma) to changes of neoplasia (as in low grade urothelial carcinoma) that, in some instances, may be distinguished from benign conditions (Figs. 3.2, 3.3). In the lowest grade lesions, nuclear crowding is the first clue that the epithelium is abnormal (Figs. 3.4–3.6).

TABLE 5. Progressive Cytologic Changes in The Grading of Urothelial Neoplasms

Diagnosis	Cytologic Criteria
Hyperplasia	cellular crowding "honeycomb" present chromatin normal umbrella cells retained
Papillary Neoplasm of Low Malignant Potential (Grade I)	chromatin coarseness loss of "honeycomb" nuclear shape elongated nuclear enlargement nucleoli indistinct umbrella cells retained
Low Grade (Grade II)	haphazard growth pattern mitoses infrequent definite increased N/C cellular enlargement uniform granular chromatin nuclear membrane irregularity homogeneous cytoplasm thickened nuclear membranes eccentric nucleus distinct nucleoli, but small umbrella cells variable
High Grade (Grade III)	large cells, often single very high N/C irregular nuclear outlines nucleoli prominent cytoplasmic differentiation, i.e. glandular/squamous variable coarse chromatin mitoses frequent umbrella cells absent

Low Grade Urothelial Carcinoma (Grade II)

Cellular Features of Low Grade Urothelial Carcinoma (Figs. 3.7–3.19)

Diagnosis	Cytologic Criteria
Low Grade	haphazard growth pattern
(Grade II)	mitoses infrequent
	definite increased N/C
	cellular enlargement
	uniform granular chromatin
	nuclear membrane irregularity
	homogeneous cytoplasm
	thickened nuclear membranes
	eccentric nucleus
	distinct nucleoli, but small
	umbrella cells variable

Using statistical analysis, the cytologic features of homogeneous cytoplasm (i.e., absence of vacuoles), increased NC ratio, and slight nuclear membrane irregularity were determined by Raab to be the most reliable features of low grade neoplasms in bladder washing specimens. Some authors have claimed that the sensitivity of detection approximates 70% if these criteria are used. For the diagnosis of low grade carcinoma in bladder washing specimens, individual cells within groups should be examined for diagnostic criteria. Discussion with the cystoscopist may establish that the lesion is a papillary tumor.

Upper Tract Lesions (Figs. 3.20, 3.21)

In the case of upper tract lesions, the problem is more challenging because the non-neoplastic epithelium may exhibit more atypical features than in voided urine. Careful consideration of IVP or retrograde films and the suspicions of the urologist will play an important role in the final decision. Considerable caution must be incorporated into any diagnosis of a low grade lesion in the upper tract because of the therapeutic implications. Loss of a kidney because of instrumentation artifact or hyperplasia originally diagnosed as a neoplasm (Fig. 3.1) is a serious consequence of interpretive error. Biopsy confirmation is clearly indicated before a nephrectomy is performed. Careful follow-up without surgery is recommended in the absence of radiographic evidence of a neoplasm in these borderline instances. Pitfalls are listed in Table 6.

TABLE 6. Mimics of Low Grade Lesions Obtained From Washings

	Low Grade	Instrumentation	Calculi
Cellularity	High	High	Low
Cytoplasm	Opaque	Textured	Frayed
Nucleus-size	Larger	Normal	Larger
Nucleus-shape	Oval, irregular	Round	Irregular
Nucleoli	Absent	Tiny	Variable
Chromatin	Uniform, darker	Pale, uniform	Very dark
N/C	Increased	Normal	Variable
Background	Clean	Clean	Dirty

High Grade Urothelial Carcinoma

Recognition of the high grade carcinomas is magnitudes easier than the lower grade lesions simply because of well-established malignant criteria that also apply to urinary tract cytology (Figs. 3.22, 3.23). When examining these cases, the cytology student (even the older ones) should take such opportunity to appreciate the subtle changes in the nuclear contour that will separate lowest grade lesions, with an oval or round shape, from the carcinomas, which have obviously irregular nuclear outlines.

Cytologic Features of High Grade Carcinoma (Figs. 3.24–3.39)

Diagnosis	Cytologic Criteria
High Grade (Grade III)	large cells, often single
	very high N/C
	irregular nuclear outlines
	nucleoli prominent
	cytoplasmic differentiation, i.e. glandular/squamous
	variable coarse chromatin
	mitoses frequent
	umbrella cells absent

In low grade carcinoma (Grade 2), monotonous neoplasia is evident even on low power. The chromatin is granular and irregularly distributed. The nuclear size increases as does the overall size of the cell. In tissue fragments, definite disorganization and occasional mitotic figures are seen. Nucleoli may be conspicuous but not necessarily enlarged. They are not requisite for diagnosis.

In high grade lesions (Grade 3), anaplasia is obvious. All of the criteria of malignancy are present: cells are enlarged and NC ratios high; nuclear chromatin is variable in texture and distribution; nucleoli are prominent. Differentiation into squamous (Fig. 3.27) and glandular cell types (Fig. 3.33) can be seen, but should not change the diagnosis from urothelial carcinoma. These "metaplasias" are characteristic of urothelium, especially when it becomes neoplastic. Even if a mucin stain is positive, this finding should be cautiously interpreted, for a urothelial carcinoma with glandular features is treated considerably differently from an adenocarcinoma of the bladder, the latter demanding a cystectomy. A high grade urothelial carcinoma can still be treated conservatively depending upon staging and clinical considerations.

Carcinoma In Situ: The Concept

"The past preoccupation with the clinically apparent exophytic papillary neoplasms may prove to be a major error in identifying the enemy, if the aggressive clinical behavior of invasive bladder carcinoma originates in flat carcinoma in situ." (R.O. Peterson: Urologic Pathology)

Our frame of reference of carcinoma in situ (CIS) unfortunately is learned in the context of the lesion arising in the uterine cervix. Cervical squamous CIS has a very long natural history (average 10 years from first neoplastic changes to carcinoma), and many of the lesions never progress to invasive disease. Such is not the case with CIS of the urinary bladder. This lesion is invariably of high grade, is more rapidly invasive (generally within three years of diagnosis of CIS), potentially fatal, and often accompanies papillary low grade lesions. Fortunately, most urologists and cytopathologists are knowledgeable about this lesion's biologic behavior, its detection and management. Koss wisely emphasizes that "carcinoma in situ is a primary target for cytologic diagnosis". While he still considers CIS as a "precursor lesion", Koss emphasizes the importance of considering the entire urinary tract as suspect for CIS whenever a lower grade papillary carcinoma is detected. He cautions that "the status of the peripheral epithelium of the bladder must be determined by cytology of the urinary sediment and by multiple biopsies... in all patients with neoplastic diseases of the bladder". Indeed, perhaps Koss's greatest contribution to pathology has been demonstrating by "bladder mapping" the various grades of urologic neoplasms that can occur simultaneously.

Therefore, in any patient, with either an historic or current bladder tumor, the cytologic sample must not only be examined to verify the obvious, the grossly visible lesion, but should be carefully scrutinized to find even a few single cells which may indicate a high grade lesion, the insidious and treacherous carcinoma in situ.

Histologic Criteria

Tissue diagnosis of the high grade sessile (flat) lesions is made difficult by the variable and often deceptive thinness of the mucosa, ranging from 3–20 cells thick. Critical to the histologic diagnosis is individual cell atypia, which correlates closely with the cytologic findings. Although WHO/ISUP terminology includes dysplastic precursor lesions, essentially equivalent to the intra-epithelial lesions of the uterine cervix, the classic CIS lesion of the urinary bladder has full thickness change consisting of significantly enlarged cells with high nuclear-cytoplasmic ratios; nuclei display hyperchromasia, irregular nuclear membranes, and disoriented polarity. Mitotic figures complete the picture. The overall impression of the urothelium is one of pleomorphic disorganization.

Because of the well-known predilection of high grade cells to easily disaggregate, biopsies may have almost no epithelial cells once they are processed. The phenomenon of "denudation" must be considered whenever such a biopsy is encountered, and a high grade lesion considered. Correlation with concurrent cytology is recommended. Our pathologists have on occasion processed the formalin in which the denuded biopsy was submitted to the laboratory and have recovered diagnostic cells.

Cytologic Criteria

As the name implies, CIS is without invasion; therefore, the background of any sample will lack blood, significant inflammation and cell debris. Cells of a CIS classically shed singly, are enlarged at least four times that of normal basal urothelial cells, have very high NC ratios, coarsely clumped chromatin, irregular nuclear outlines, and often prominent nucleoli (Figs. 3.36–3.39). They are morphologically more similar to squamous cells than to urothelial cells.

When the sample is obtained by catheterization or washing, tissue fragments may be present, and these should be carefully examined to appreciate the enlarged nuclear size, the increased NC ratios, and the other features mentioned above, as well as disorganized growth (Figs. 3.30, 3.31). The clean background will confirm the lack of invasion, the cytologic details of the cells will provide the high grade, the combination of which defines "carcinoma in situ".

Invasive High Grade Carcinoma (Figs. 3.40–3.43)

Invasion cannot be reliably predicted since blood and inflammatory debris may be seen with benign cystitis as well as invasive carcinoma (Figs. 3.40, 3.41). Both in situ and invasive urothelial carcinoma have essentially identical cytologic criteria. Rarely, spindle cells reminiscent of the "fiber cells" of invasive squamous carcinoma of the cervix will be noted, but this feature is infrequent enough to be of no practical use (Figs. 3.42, 3.43). Biopsy is necessary to determine involvement of detrusor muscle invasion that cannot be predicted by any cytomorphologic criteria.

Mimics of High Grade Carcinoma (Table 7)

Polyoma Virus (Figs. 3.44–3.52)

The most frequently encountered cellular mimic of high grade urothelial carcinoma is produced by infection with polyoma (BK) virus. Infection can occur in otherwise healthy people, but more commonly is seen in immunocompromised patients, especially renal transplant and HIV infected individuals. When the virus infects patients with high grade bladder cancer, the diagnosis of both or either can be extremely difficult. If the sample is heavily populated with apparently infected cells and cancer cells, immunochemical staining with SV-40 antibody will mark the nuclei of infected cells (Fig. 3.51), leaving the unmarked atypical cells as a separate population, presumably from the high grade carcinoma. However, recent evidence points to polyoma virus as a potential causative agent in high grade bladder cancer. Therefore, in any patient with persistent changes of polyoma virus, a thorough work-up for urothelial carcinoma is prudent.

Urinary Calculi (also see Chapter 4)

Another cause of diagnostic confusion is calculus disease (lithiasis), as stones may create cellular changes that closely resemble neoplasia. The most robust distinguishing feature is the lack of well preserved abnormal cells when only calculus is present. Bladder washing can provide well preserved cells which may answer the question.

Further adding to the dilemma is the high rate of concurrent calculi and carcinoma, especially in the renal pelvis. When in doubt, caution is prudent. Since clinicians don't always appreciate the importance of providing the cytopathologist with stone history, education is warranted whenever the occasion arises.

TABLE 7. Mimics of High Grade Lesions Obtained From Washings

	High grade	Reactive	Calculi	Polyoma Virus	Post Therapy
Cellularity	High	Modest	Medium	Variable	Variable
Cytoplasm	Variable	Abundant	Frayed	Scant	Variable
Nucleus-size	Large	Increased	Variable	Large	Large
Nucleus-shape	Irregular	Round, oval	Irregular	Round	Irregular
Nucleoli	Variable	Prominent	Variable	Absent	Prominent
Chromatin	Dark, irregular	Granular, uniform	Dark, coarse	Ground glass, marginated	Variable, dark
N/C	High	Moderate	Variable	High	Moderate
Background	Variable	Inflamed	Dirty	Variable	Inflamed

Low Grade Urothelial Lesions 67

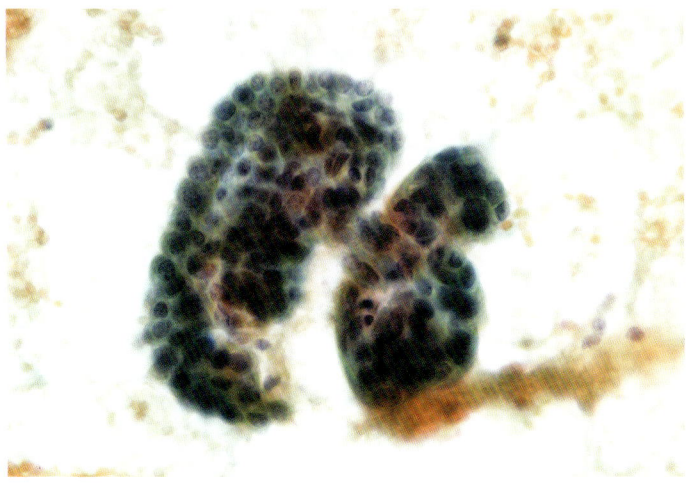

FIGURE 3.1. Hyperplasia—renal pelvic brushing: Massive hematuria brought a 35 year old woman to the emergency department. Urograms disclosed a "mass" in the renal pelvis of one kidney. This brushing was considered to be consistent with a low grade papillary carcinoma. Nephrectomy revealed the source of her bleeding to be rupture of a sub-mucosal hemangioma in the renal pelvis. The "mass" was a blood clot. Urothelium nearby was hyperplastic, the source of these fragments. Note the round uniform small nuclei, orderly arrangement, and adequate cytoplasm. (400x)

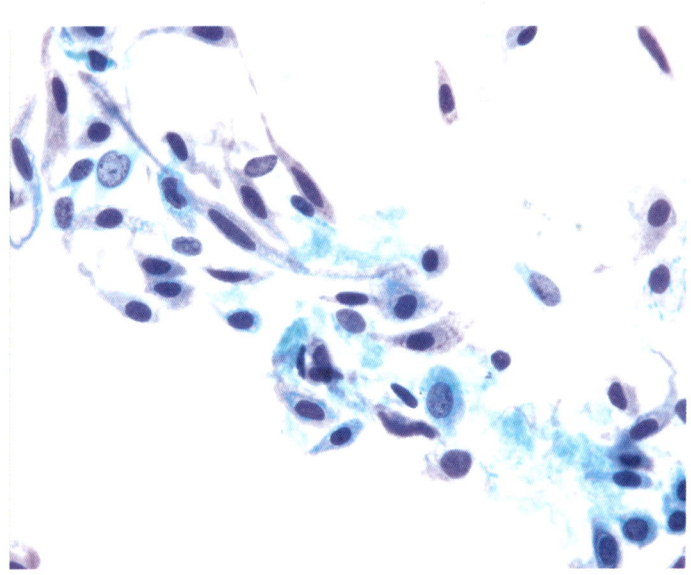

FIGURE 3.2. Papillary Urothelial Neoplasm of Low Malignant Potential—renal pelvic brushing: Numerous elongated columnar cells, many with bi-polar cytoplasmic extensions, populate this unusual sample. Nuclear chromatin is slightly darker than that of the rare umbrella cells in the picture and homogeneous. The oval nuclei have smooth and thin nuclear borders. Nucleoli are absent in the tumor cells, but obvious in the umbrella cells. (400x)

Low Grade Urothelial Lesions 69

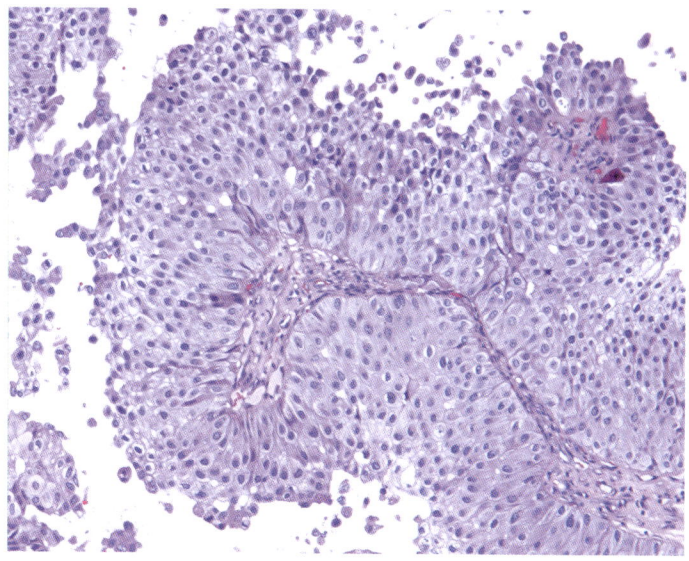

FIGURE 3.3. Low Grade Papillary Carcinoma—bladder biopsy: Papillary architecture is supported on a fibrovascular stalk. The overall organization is orderly, nuclear size and NC ratios are relatively uniform and no mitotic figures are seen. (H&E, 100x)

70   3. Grading Urothelial Neoplasms

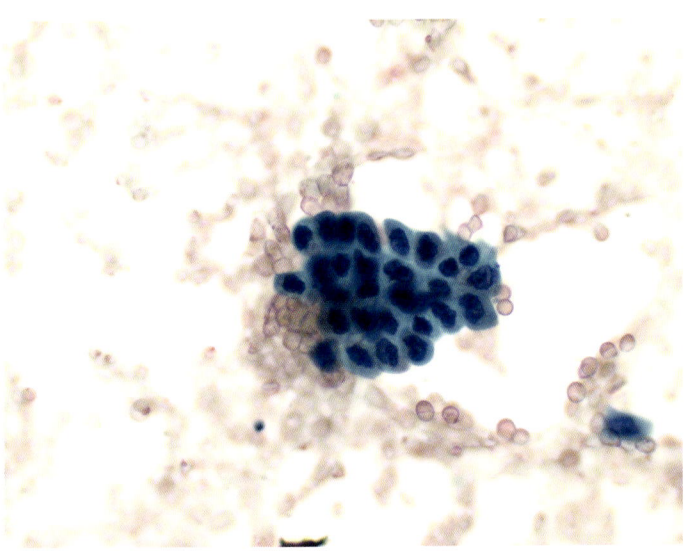

FIGURE 3.4. Low Grade Urothelial Carcinoma—bladder washing: The neoplastic cells exhibit increased nuclear to cytoplasmic ratios and homogeneous cytoplasm. The nuclei are slightly more hyperchromatic than usually observed in low grade carcinomas, and the nuclear membrane irregularities are pronounced. (600x)

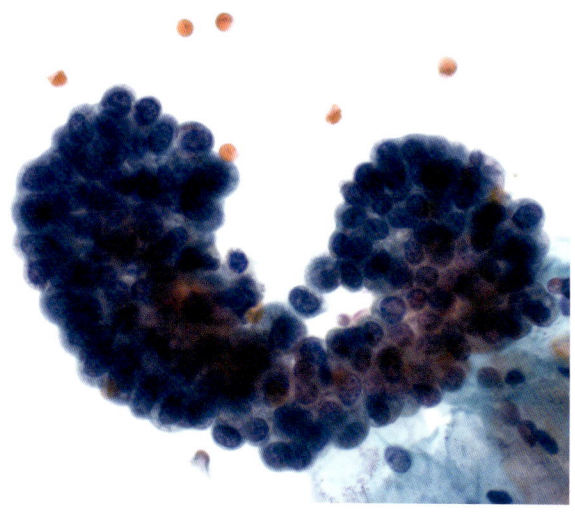

FIGURE 3.5. Low Grade Urothelial Carcinoma—catheterized urine: A 3-dimensional pseudopapillary cluster of neoplastic cells is seen. The cells show a hobnail appearance at the edge and an absence of umbrella cells, although umbrella cells may be attached, in other cases, to a low grade urothelial carcinoma cluster. The cells have an increased nuclear to cytoplasmic ratio, although the nuclei are not significantly larger than intermediate squamous cell nuclei. In this case, the nuclei appear moderately hyperchromatic and the nuclear membranes are thickened. (600x)

72   3. Grading Urothelial Neoplasms

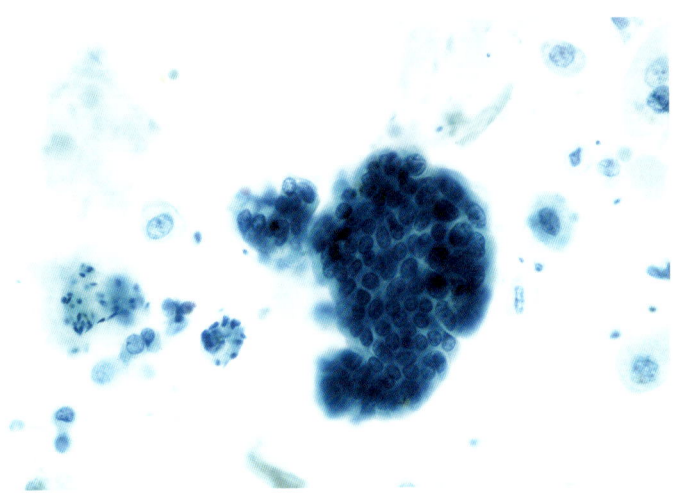

FIGURE 3.6. Low Grade Papillary Carcinoma—bladder washing: The cellular changes of low grade lesions are minimal, one of the difficulties in diagnosing these lesions. Architectural crowding with minimal nuclear atypia are the most robust features. (400x)

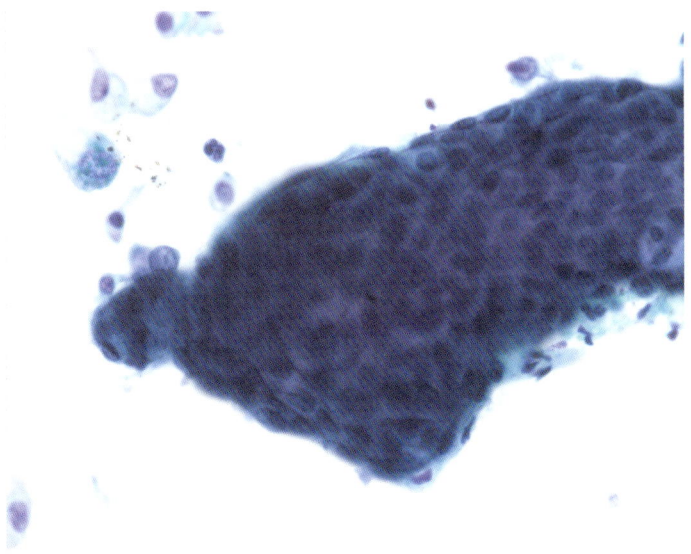

FIGURE 3.7. Low Grade Papillary Carcinoma—bladder washing: A papillary fragment with smooth boundaries contains cells with nuclei that are relatively small, uniform in size, and frequently oval. Although this fragment is quite thick, a transparent stain and careful focusing will enable appreciation of the nuclear crowding characteristic of a low grade lesion. (400x)

74   3. Grading Urothelial Neoplasms

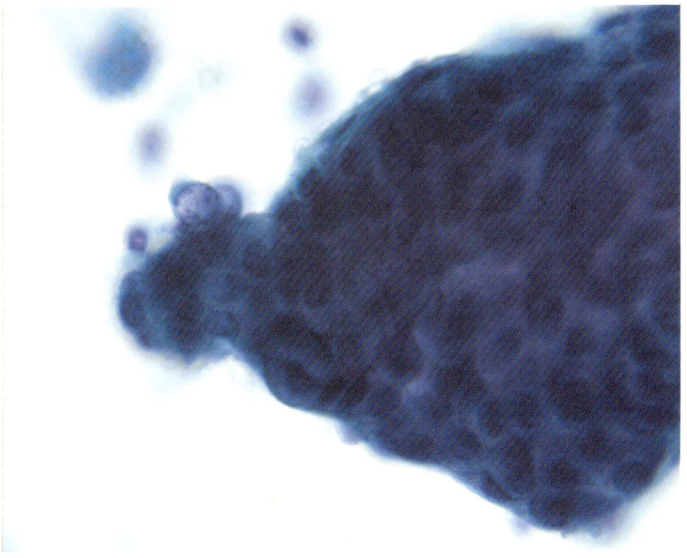

FIGURE 3.8. Low Grade Papillary Carcinoma—bladder washing: A true tissue fragment consists of cells with relatively low NC ratios and uniformly round nuclei. The papillary architecture is verified by the smooth boundary of the fragment, not to be confused with an instrumented sheet of urothelial cells (see Figure 2.10). (600x)

Low Grade Urothelial Carcinoma 75

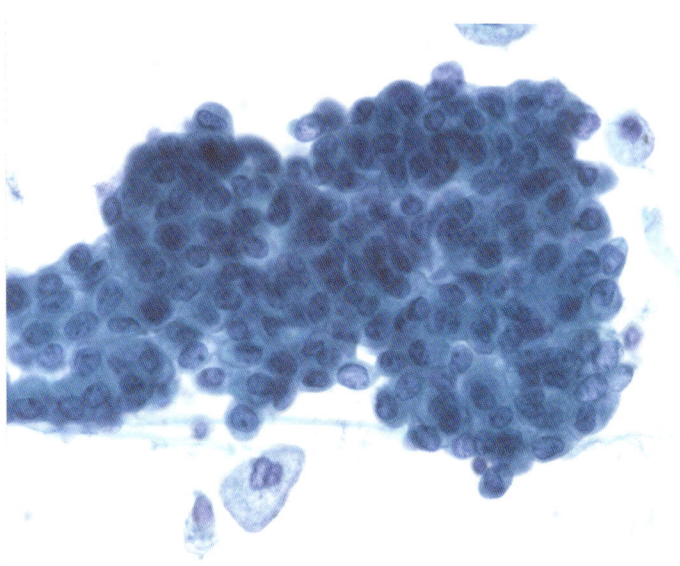

FIGURE 3.9. Low grade Papillary Carcinoma—bladder washing: Polarity is lost as nuclei are oriented in various directions in these tissue fragments with disorganized architecture. Nuclear sizes vary as well as nuclear shapes. Many nuclei have longitudinal grooves and pinpoint nucleoli. The small nuclear size (compare with urothelial cells in the bottom of the photograph) and nuclear overlapping are additional criteria of a low grade malignancy. (400x)

76   3. Grading Urothelial Neoplasms

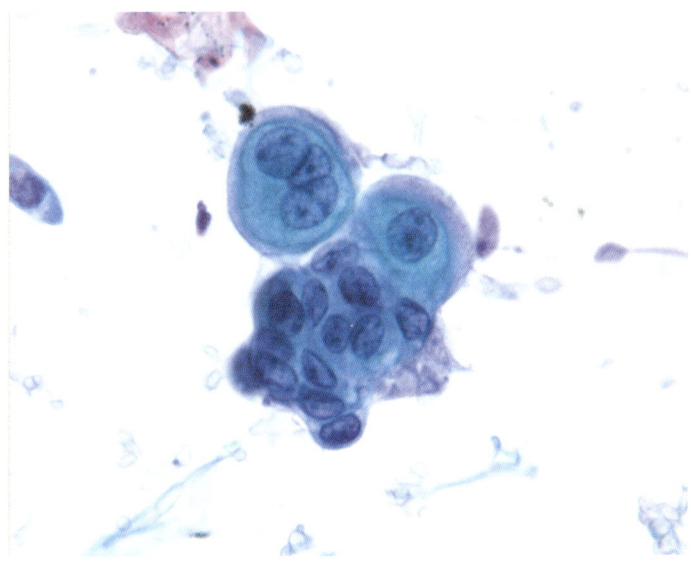

FIGURE 3.10. Low Grade Urothelial Carcinoma—bladder washing: Two umbrella cells in the upper portion of the photograph can be contrasted with the tissue fragment in the lower field. The benign umbrella cells have round nuclei, whereas the tumor fragment is characterized by nuclear overlapping and oval nuclear shape. Several tumor cells also have longitudinal nuclear grooves. (600x)

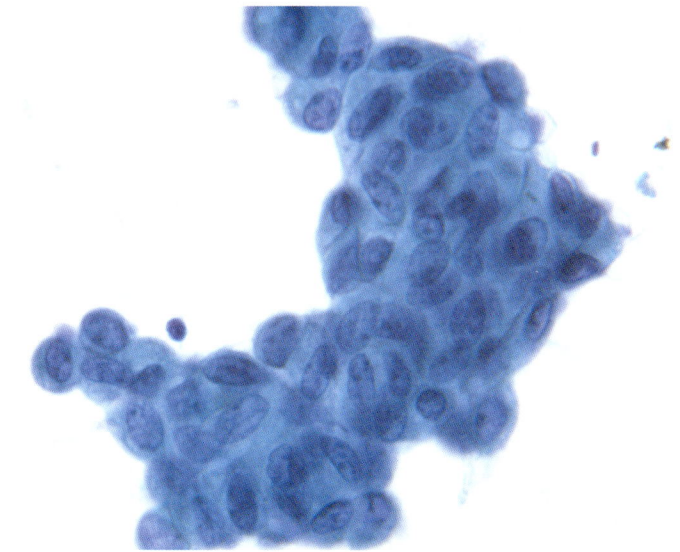

FIGURE 3.11. Low Grade Papillary Carcinoma—bladder washing: Characteristic is the disorderly architecture and oval nuclei with occasional longitudinal nuclear grooves. Chromatin is relatively bland and nucleoli, if present, are indistinct. (600x)

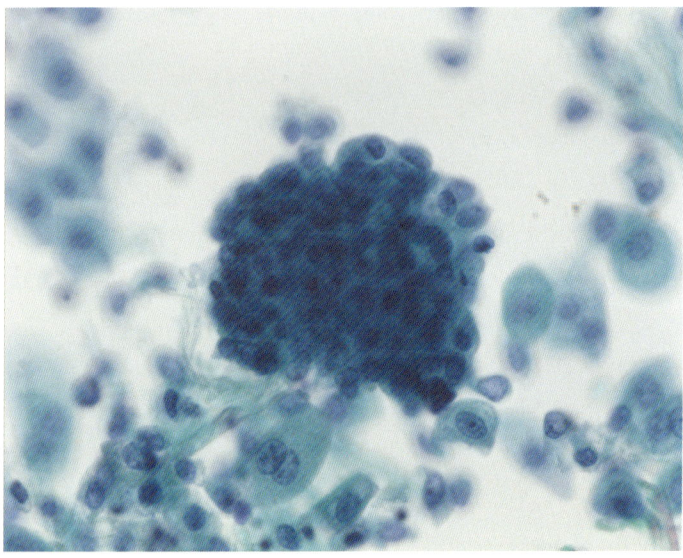

FIGURE 3.12. Low Grade Papillary Carcinoma—bladder washing: Although instrumentation can produce fragments of tissue, the architecture is the reliable diagnostic feature. Note the crowding of cells, the high NC ratios and the nuclear overlapping. The nuclei are small when compared with those of the umbrella cells in the lower portion of the photograph. (400x).

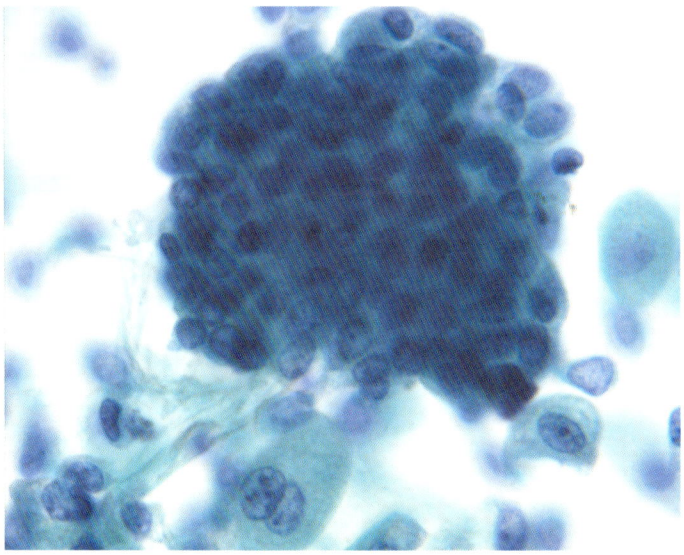

FIGURE 3.13. Low Grade Papillary Carcinoma—bladder washing: The architecture of a fragment of urothelial cells is disorganized with nuclear overlapping and crowding. However, the nuclei are small and chromatin is relatively even when compared with the benign urothelial cells in the lower portions of the photograph. (600x)

80   3. Grading Urothelial Neoplasms

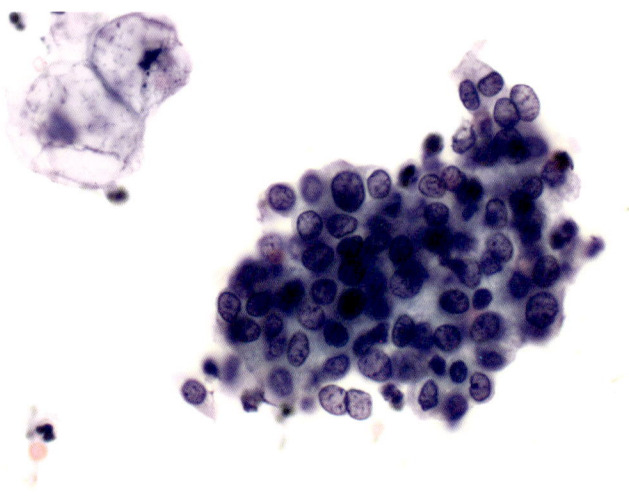

FIGURE 3.14. Low Grade Urothelial Carcinoma—bladder washing: The malignant cells exhibit mild to moderate atypia. The nuclei are slightly enlarged compared to the intermediate squamous cell nuclei seen in the upper left. The nuclear membranes are thickened, although many of the nuclei appear hypochromatic. The cytoplasm varies from homogeneous to slightly frothy. The extensive nuclear overlap also is suggestive of a low grade urothelial carcinoma, rather than reactive change. (600x)

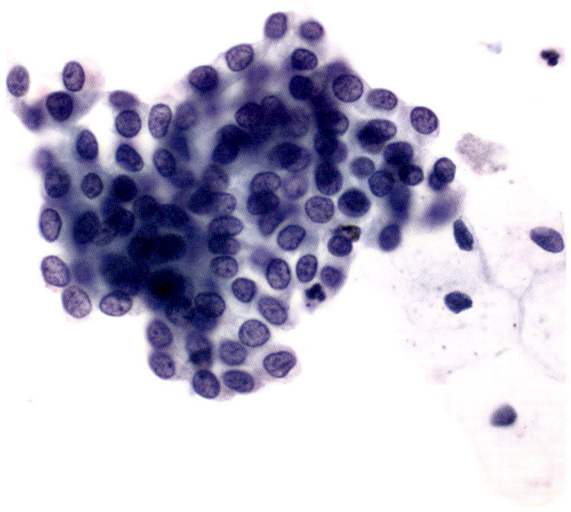

FIGURE 3.15. Low Grade Urothelial Carcinoma—catheterized urine: The neoplastic cells have a uniform appearance, and the nuclear membranes are thickened. The nuclear chromatin is hypo to only mildly hyperchromatic. The cytoplasm has a homogeneous appearance. The nuclei appear only equal to or slightly larger in size than the intermediate squamous cell nuclei. (600x)

82   3. Grading Urothelial Neoplasms

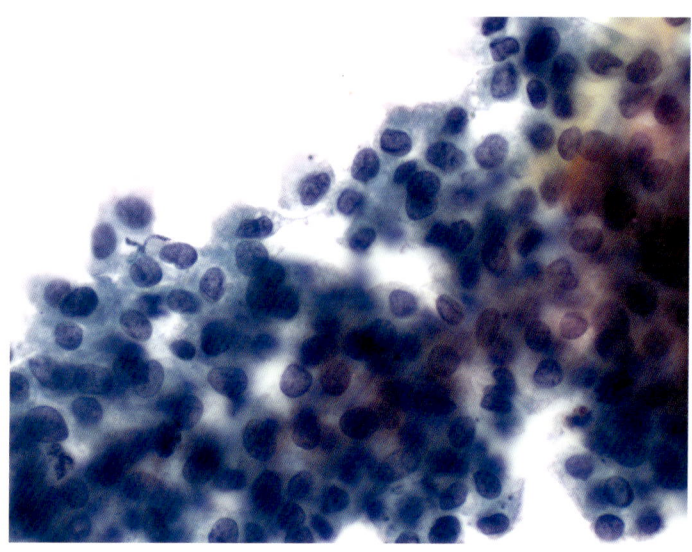

FIGURE 3.16. Low Grade Urothelial Carcinoma—bladder washing: The malignant cells have round to oval nuclei and nuclear hypochromasia. Occasional nuclei exhibit longitudinal grooves and small nucleoli. The cytoplasm has a granular appearance, although at the edges of the large fragment, cytoplasmic homogeneity is seen. Extensive nuclear overlap is present. (600x)

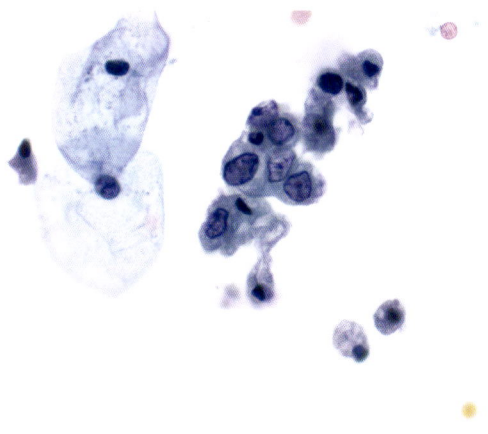

FIGURE 3.17. Low Grade Urothelial Carcinoma—voided urine: Extensive nuclear and cytoplasmic degeneration may be seen in the low grade urothelial carcinoma in voided urines. In this case, the cells appear slightly more atypical than the usual low grade urothelial carcinoma and some of this atypia may be secondary to the degenerative process. However, the cells, for the most part, do not display nuclear hyperchromasia except for the cells that have degenerated. The cytoplasm appears stringy and slightly less homogeneous than usual. The nuclear membranes are irregular in contour. (600x)

84   3. Grading Urothelial Neoplasms

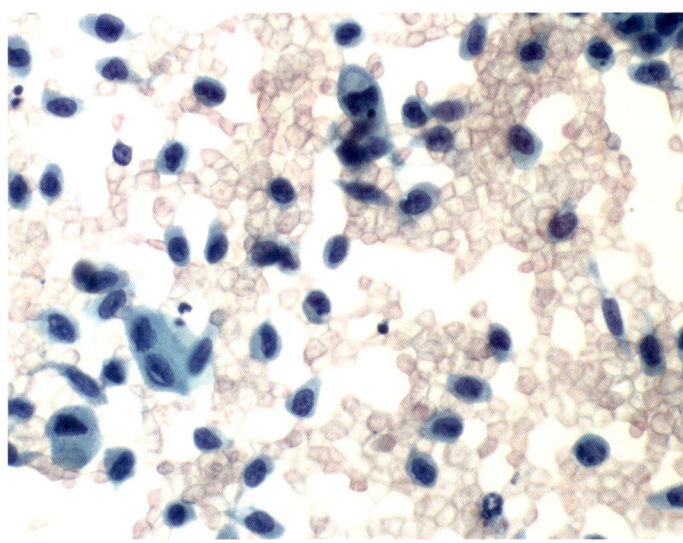

FIGURE 3.18. Low Grade Urothelial Carcinoma—bladder washing: In some low grade urothelial carcinomas, extensive cellular dissociation and degeneration is seen. In this case the cells are small, and the cells exhibit homogeneous cytoplasm and eccentrically placed nuclei. The nuclei exhibit only mild nuclear membrane irregularities. Several elongated and spindled nuclei are seen. (600x)

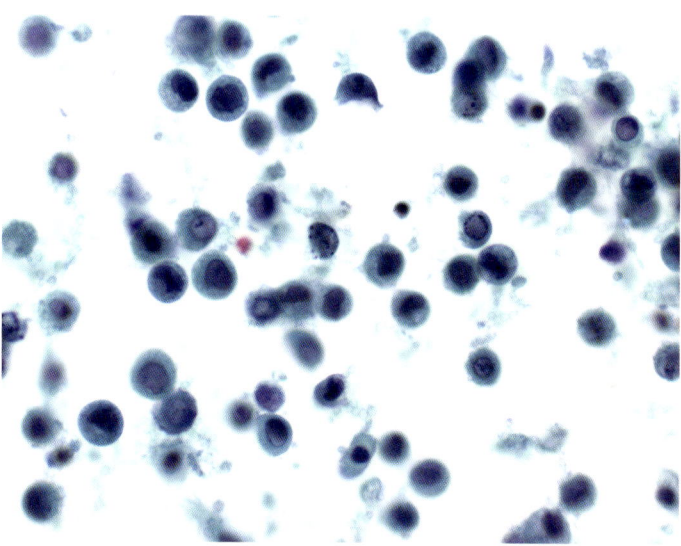

FIGURE 3.19. Low Grade Urothelial Carcinoma—bladder washing: Extensive degeneration and cellular dissociation is present. The more intact low grade carcinoma cells do not show markedly atypical nuclei and exhibit only minimal nuclear membrane irregularities and pale to slightly darkened chromatin. (600x)

86 3. Grading Urothelial Neoplasms

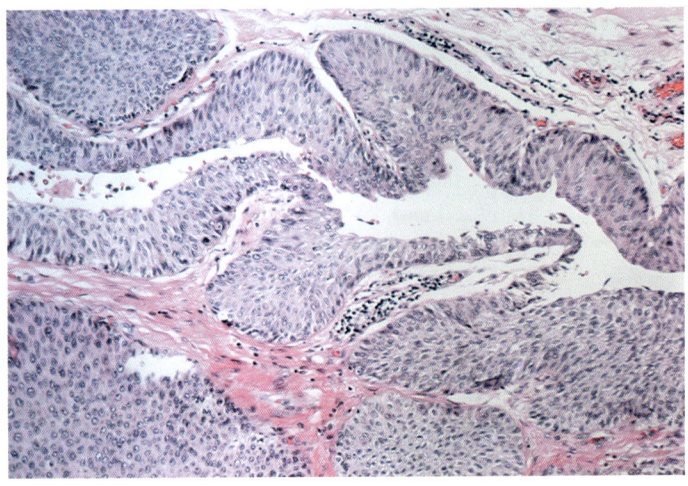

FIGURE 3.20. Low Grade Urothelial Carcinoma—ureteral biopsy: The thickened urothelium lines the ureter in an orderly fashion, but with atypical cells, consistent with a low grade lesion. Loss of umbrella cells, high NC ratios, and mild hyperchromasia are characteristic of this lesion. (H&E, 200x)

Low Grade Urothelial Carcinoma 87

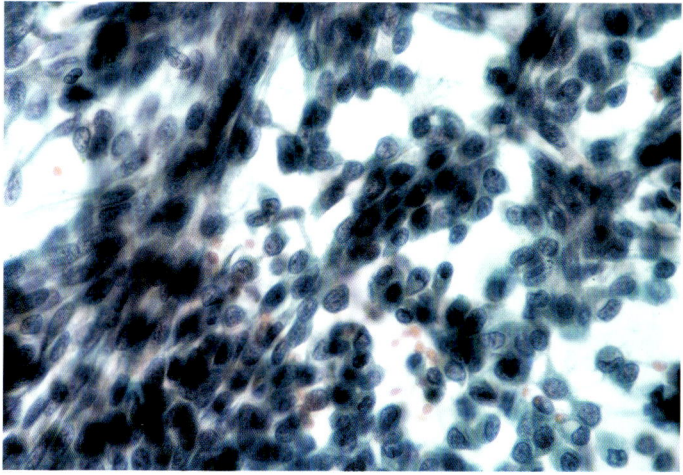

FIGURE 3.21. Low Grade Urothelial Carcinoma—ureteral brush: Cytologic diagnosis of extra-vesical urothelial lesions relys on the same criteria as lesions of the bladder. However, caution must be employed since the consequences of a false positive may result in loss of a kidney or at least major surgery. (400x)

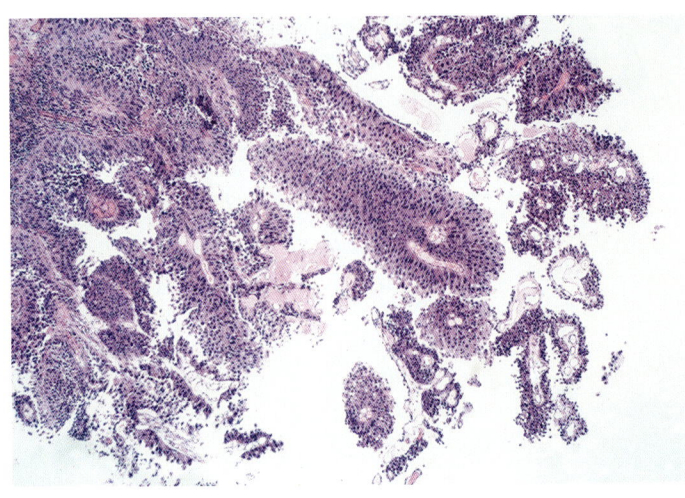

FIGURE 3.22. High Grade Papillary Urothelial Carcinoma—bladder biopsy: Although the delicate papillary architecure is more suggestive of a low grade lesion, the cellular features place this lesion in a high Grade category. (H&E, 100x)

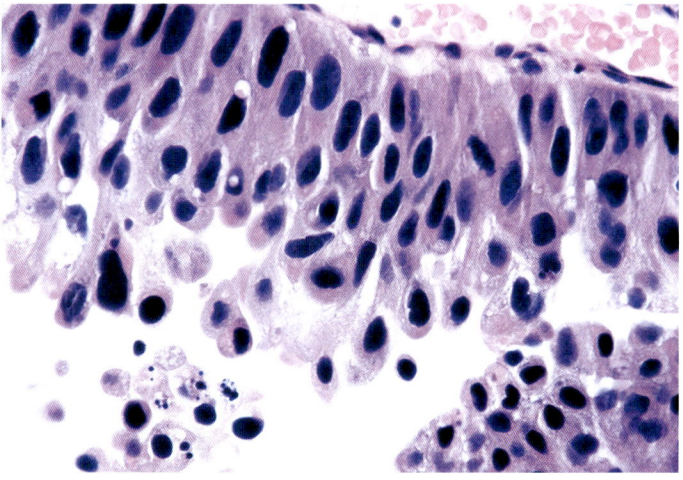

FIGURE 3.23. High Grade Papillary Urothelial Carcinoma—bladder biopsy: Higher magnification of 3.22 displays the characteristic features of high grade carcinoma, especially the high NC ratios and nuclear hyperchromasia. (H&E, 400x)

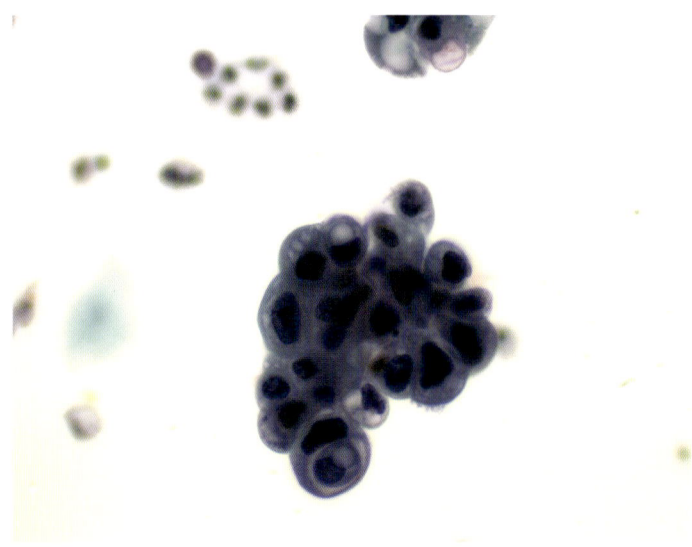

FIGURE 3.24. High Grade Urothelial Carcinoma—bladder washing: A cluster of malignant high grade urothelial cells is seen. Some malignant cells have engulfed other malignant cells and show marked nuclear hyperchromasia. Cytoplasmic vacuolization, although not prominent, may be seen in high grade urothelial carcinomas. In this case, there is not marked nuclear overlap. (600x)

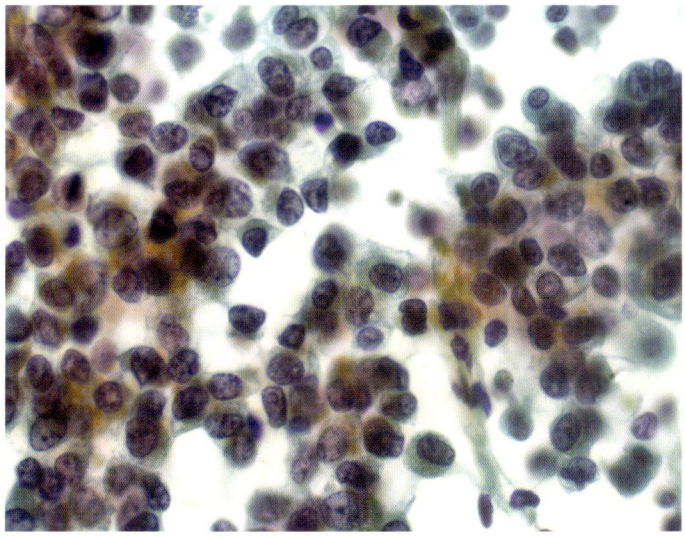

FIGURE 3.25. High Grade Urothelial Carcinoma—bladder washing: In this photomicrograph, numerous malignant cells are seen. The cells exhibit high nuclear to cytoplasmic ratios, nuclear hyperchromasia and nuclear membrane irregularities. The nuclear membrane appears thick in many instances. (600x)

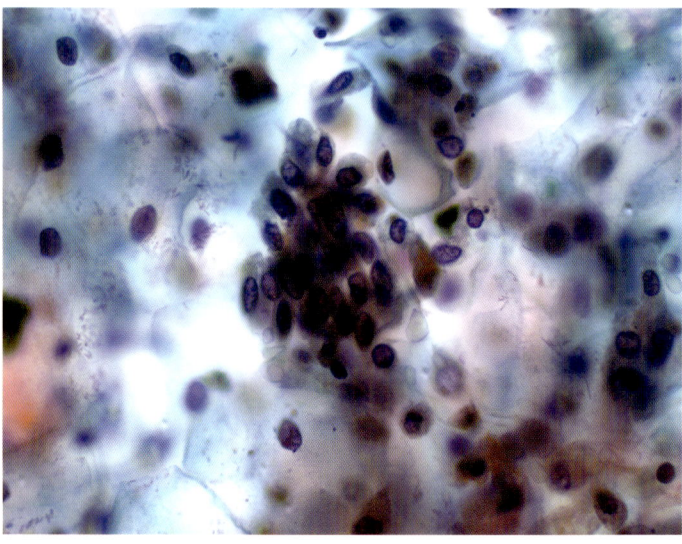

FIGURE 3.26. High Grade Urothelial Carcinoma—voided urine: Degenerated malignant cells are seen admixed with benign squamous cells. Although the nuclei are small and slightly degenerated, the nuclear membranes are markedly thickened and irregular. Often, degeneration may limit interpretation of high grade urothelial carcinoma. (600x)

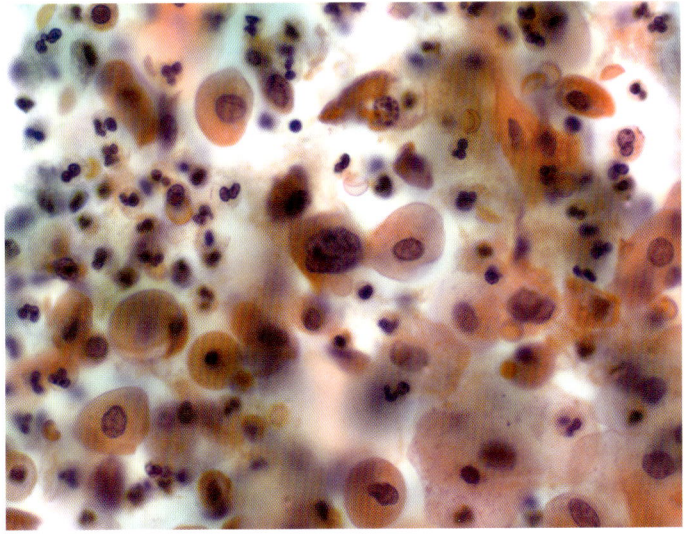

FIGURE 3.27. High Grade Urothelial Carcinoma—bladder washing: A large malignant cell is seen in the center field. Admixed are numerous neutrophils, benign urothelial cells and atypical squamous cells. In this high grade urothelial carcinoma, squamous differentiation is seen. The cytoplasm has a keratinized quality. Some types of high grade urothelial carcinomas may exhibit more pronounced squamous differentiation and may be difficult to separate from squamous carcinomas. (600x)

3. Grading Urothelial Neoplasms

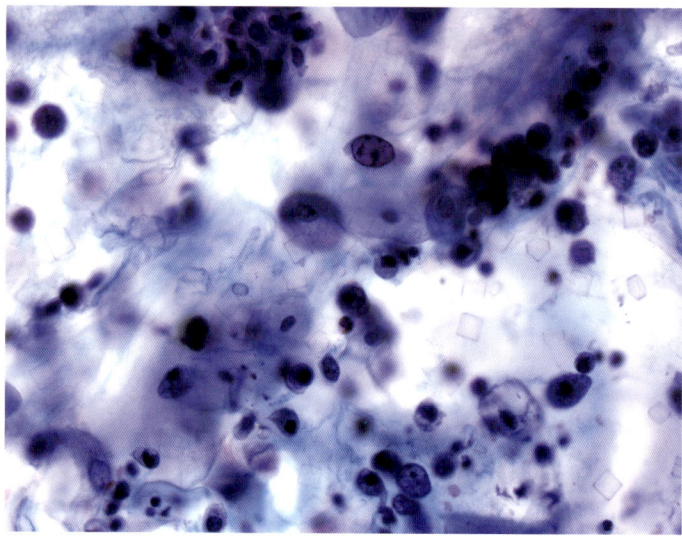

FIGURE 3.28. High Grade Urothelial Carcinoma—bladder washing: Single malignant cells are seen. These cells have high nuclear to cytoplasmic ratios and thickened nuclear membranes. Several of the cells show stripped nuclei. Numerous degenerated cells, crystals, squamous cells and debris are present in the background. (600x)

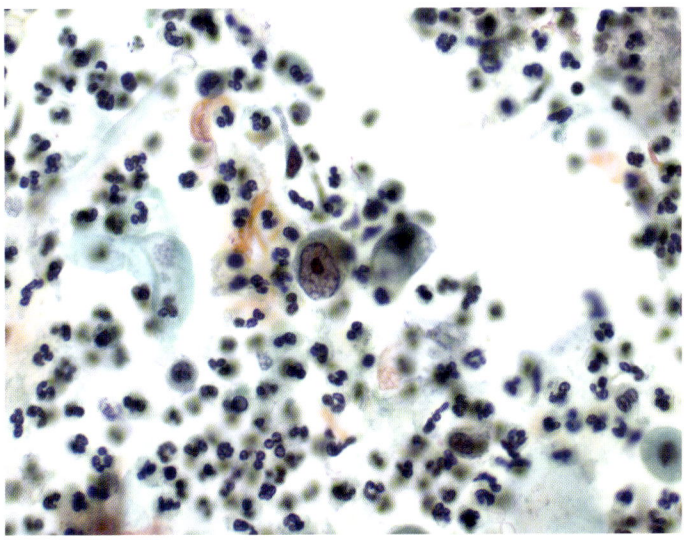

FIGURE 3.29. High Grade Urothelial Carcinoma—catheterized urine: A single neoplastic cell is seen in the center field. Some types of high grade urothelial carcinomas show prominent nucleoli and less hyperchromatic nuclei. In this case, abundant acute inflammation is admixed with debris. The neoplastic cell has an enlarged nucleus and a high nuclear to cytoplasmic ratio. (600x)

96 3. Grading Urothelial Neoplasms

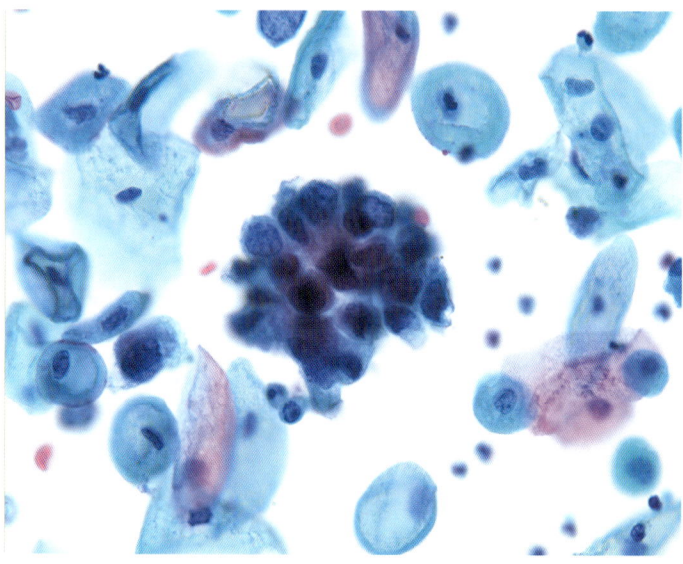

FIGURE 3.30. High Grade Urothelial Carcinoma—bladder washing: A true tissue fragment in the center is composed of primitive epithelial cells with high NC ratios and irregular nuclear outlines. Nuclear chromatin is granular and nuclear shapes are variable. Compare these cells with surrounding benign squamous and urothelial cells. (400x)

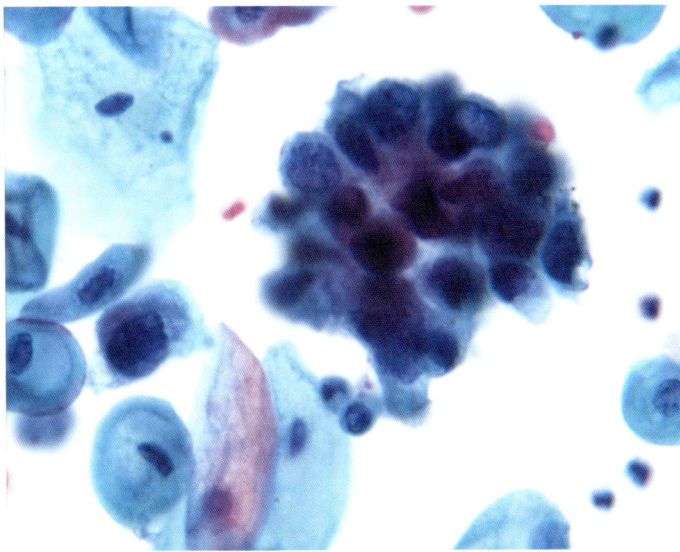

FIGURE 3.31. High Grade Urothelial Carcinoma—bladder washing: A true tissue fragment consists of enlarged cells with high NC ratios. The nuclear outlines are irregular as are the shapes. Chromatin is granular. Compare with surrounding normal squamous and urothelial cells at the periphery of the photograph. (600x)

98   3. Grading Urothelial Neoplasms

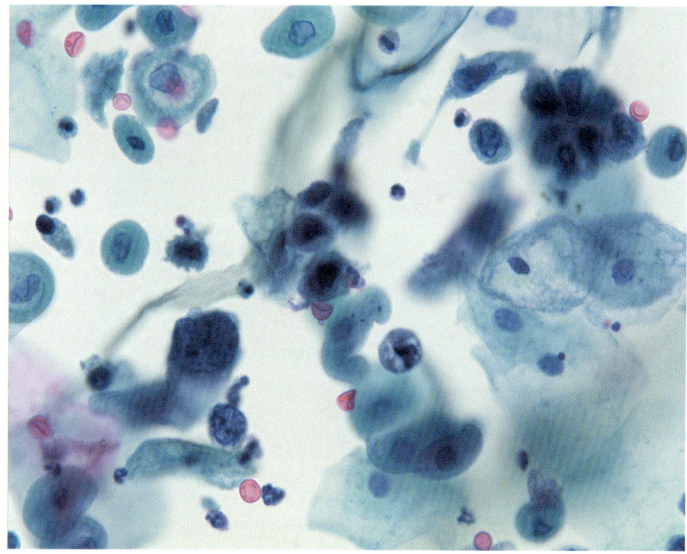

FIGURE 3.32. High Grade Urothelial Carcinoma—bladder washing: Cells display characteristic variation in cellular size, NC ratio, cytoplasmic shapes and nuclear irregularity. Contrast the obvious malignant cells with the smaller cells with low NC ratios. (400x)

High Grade Urothelial Carcinoma   99

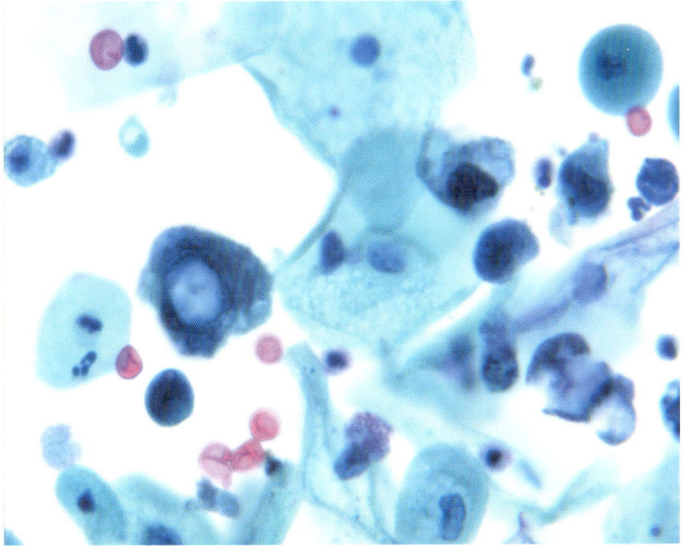

FIGURE 3.33. High Grade Urothelial Carcinoma—voided urine: High grade lesions present with a variety of cellular features, including cytoplasmic vacuolization. Unless the cellular changes are consistently those of an adenocarcinoma, such vacuoles should not persuade against the diagnosis of high grade urothelial carcinoma. Other cells in this photograph do not have vacuolated cytoplasm and are characteristic of high grade urothelial malignancy. (600x)

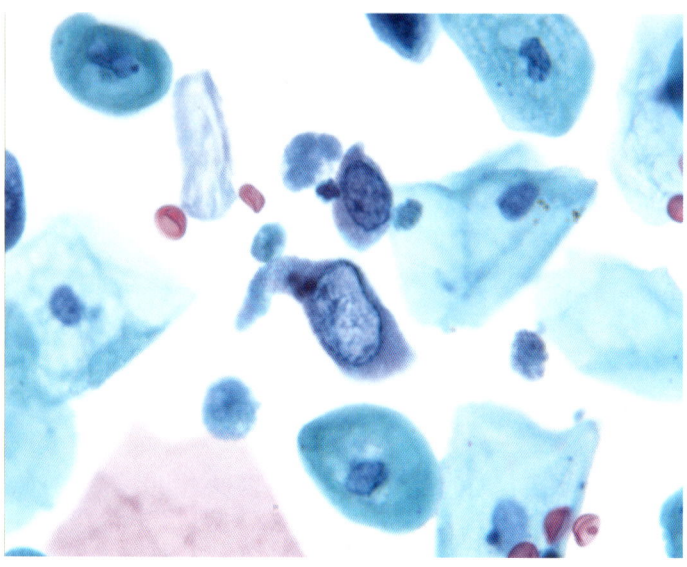

FIGURE 3.34. High Grade Urothelial Carcinoma—bladder washing: Individual cells have high NC ratios, irregular nuclear shapes and overall cellular enlargement. The nuclear chromatin is unevenly distributed. Compare with surrounding benign squamous and urothelial cells. (600x)

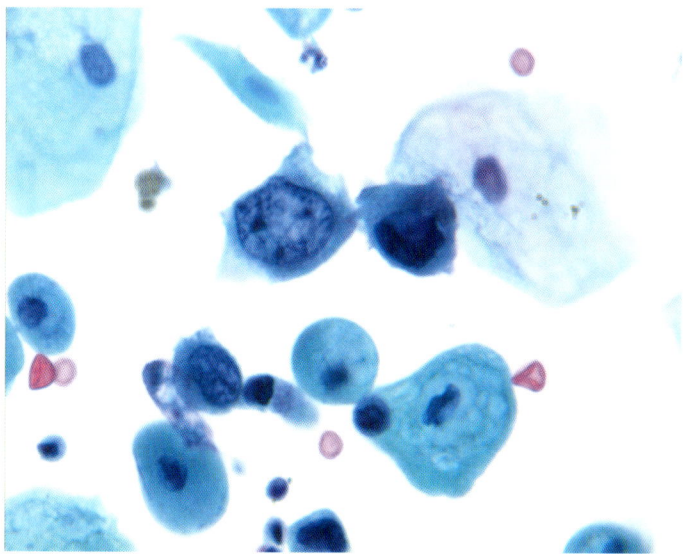

FIGURE 3.35. High Grade Urothelial Carcinoma—bladder washing: Several very large malignant cells display varying sizes, nuclear shapes, and chromatin distribution. The cell in the center right could be infected with polyoma virus, but its irregular nuclear shape is diagnostic of a cancer cell rather than a benign decoy cell. (600x)

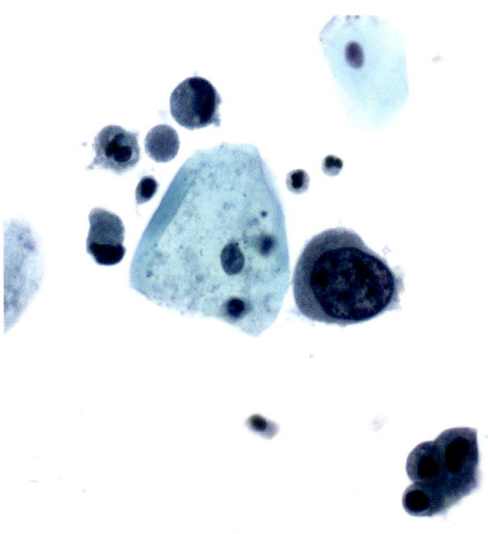

FIGURE 3.36. High Grade Urothelial Carcinoma—voided urine: Voided urine specimens may show few malignant cells that exhibit extensive degeneration. In this case, a large malignant cell is seen in the center of the field. The cell has an eccentric nucleus, and the nuclear chromatin is hyperchromatic and does not have the appearance of the nuclei seen in cells infected with human polyoma virus. (600x)

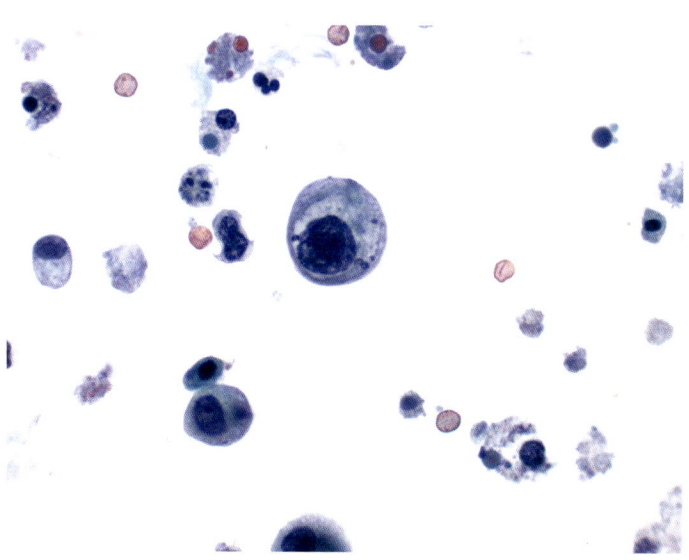

FIGURE 3.37. High Grade Urothelial Carcinoma—voided urine: Several malignant cells are seen in this photomicrograph, although the largest malignant cell is seen in the center. The nuclear to cytoplasmic ratio is not markedly increased, although the nucleus is hyperchromatic and has an irregular nuclear membrane. The cytoplasm is variegated. The nuclear size is huge compared to red blood cells and acute inflammatory cells are seen in the background. (600x)

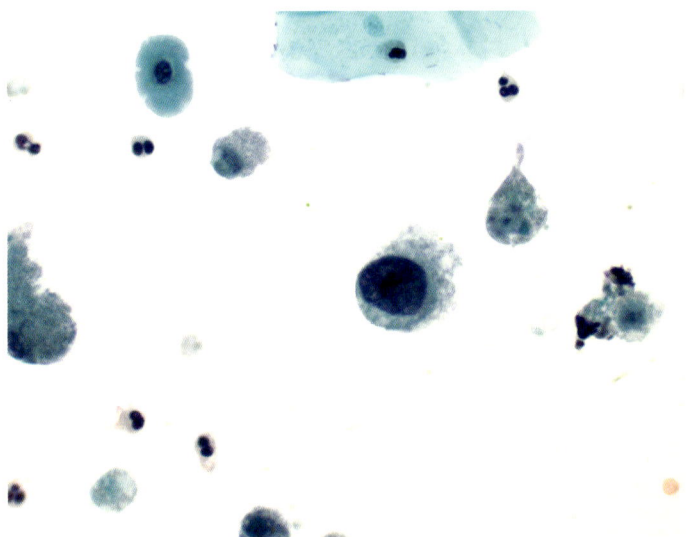

FIGURE 3.38. High Grade Urothelial Carcinoma—voided urine: A malignant urothelial cell is seen in the center field. The nucleus is hyperchromatic and has a slightly irregular nuclear membrane. Compared to the benign urothelial cell nuclei, the nucleus is huge. The cytoplasm is frothy and slightly degenerated and an acute inflammatory background is seen. In voided specimens, only a few malignant cells may be observed. (600x)

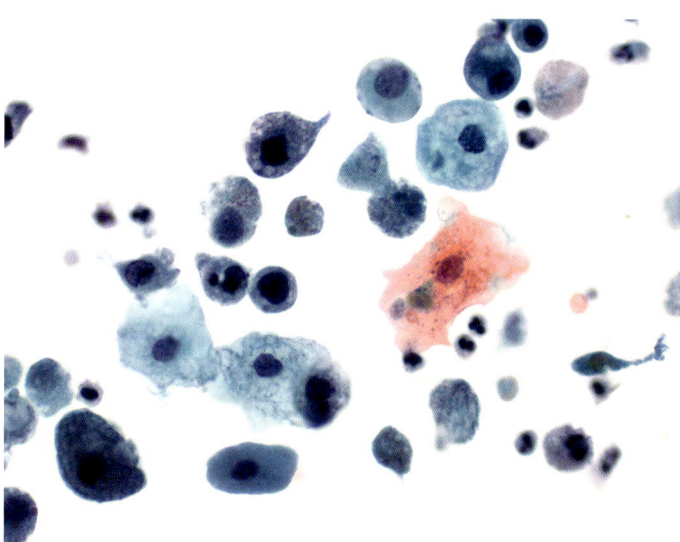

FIGURE 3.39. High Grade Urothelial Carcinoma—bladder washing: In this bladder washing specimen, numerous degenerated malignant cells are seen. In some cases of urothelial carcinoma, only few intact non-degenerated malignant cells are seen. These cells exhibit marked nuclear hyperchromasia and slightly increased nuclear to cytoplasmic ratios. A background of acute inflammation and several benign squamous cells are observed. (600x)

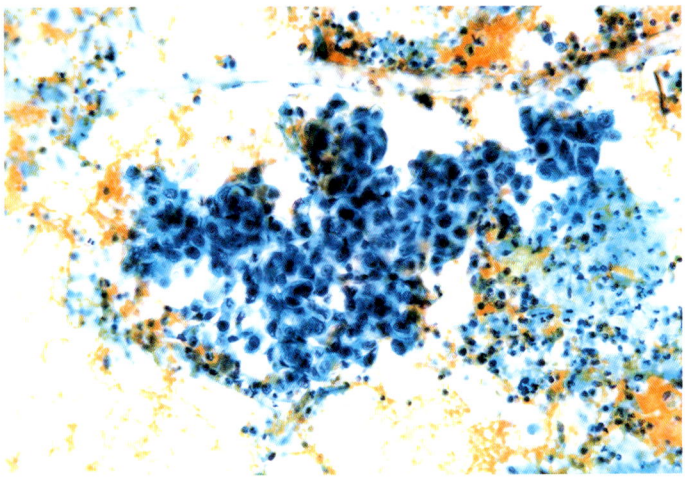

FIGURE 3.40. Invasive High Grade Urothelial Carcinoma—bladder washing: Against a background of blood and inflammation, groups of tumor cells suggest an invasive lesion. Such blood and debris are not universally an indicater of invasion in bladder lesions in contrast to the "tumor diathesis" of cervical cancer. (200x)

High Grade Urothelial Carcinoma 107

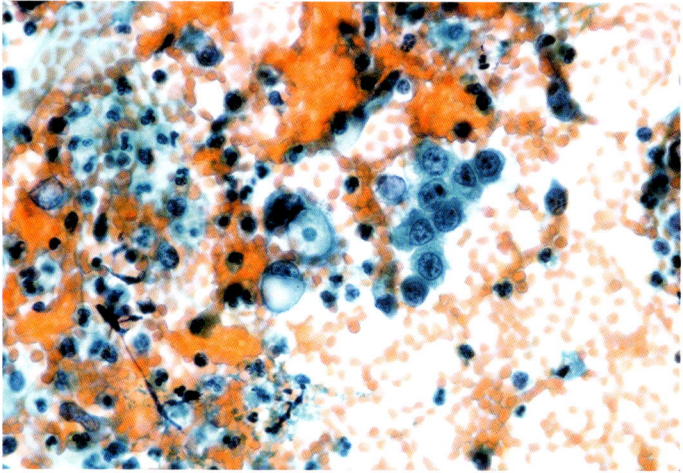

FIGURE 3.41. Invasive Urothelial Carcinoma—bladder washing: Without diagnostic tumor cells, a diagnosis of malignancy should not be made despite the debris and blood in the background. (400x)

108   3. Grading Urothelial Neoplasms

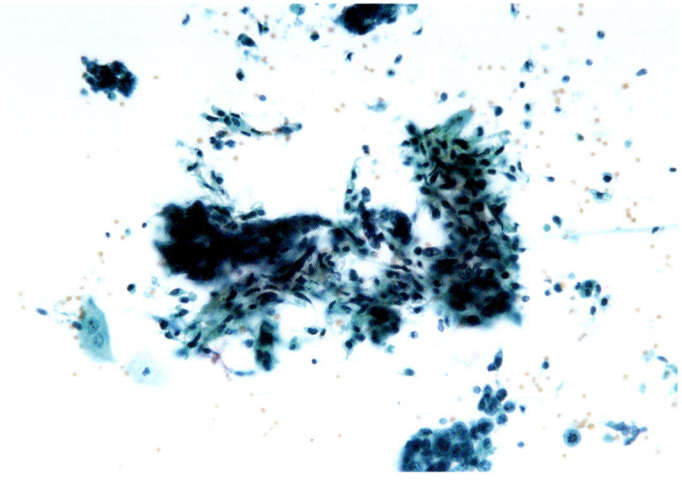

FIGURE 3.42. Invasive High Grade Urothelial Carcinoma—bladder washing: Malignant spindle or fiber cells are one of the hallmarks of invasive squamous carcinoma of the uterine cervix. Rarely seen in bladder cancer, when present these cells are also indicative of invasion. Unfortunately, the infrequency of this finding makes it of low utility. (200x)

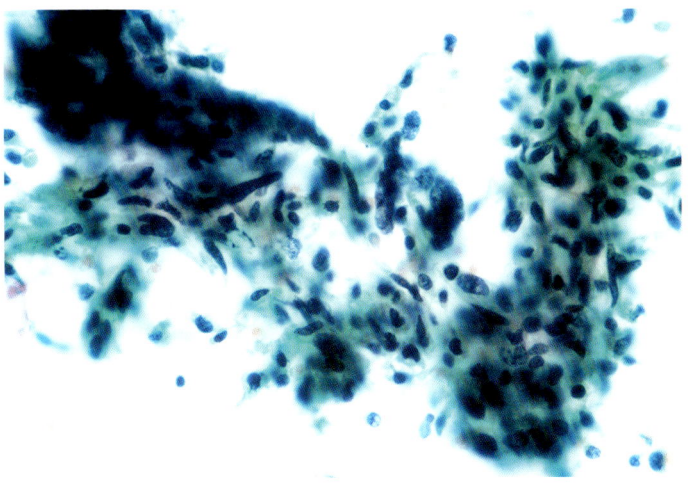

FIGURE 3.43. Invasive High Grade Urothelial Carcinoma—bladder washing: Higher magnification of 3.42 verifies the malignant characteristics of the fiber cells and the accompanying larger tumor cells. Note the relatively clean background. (400x)

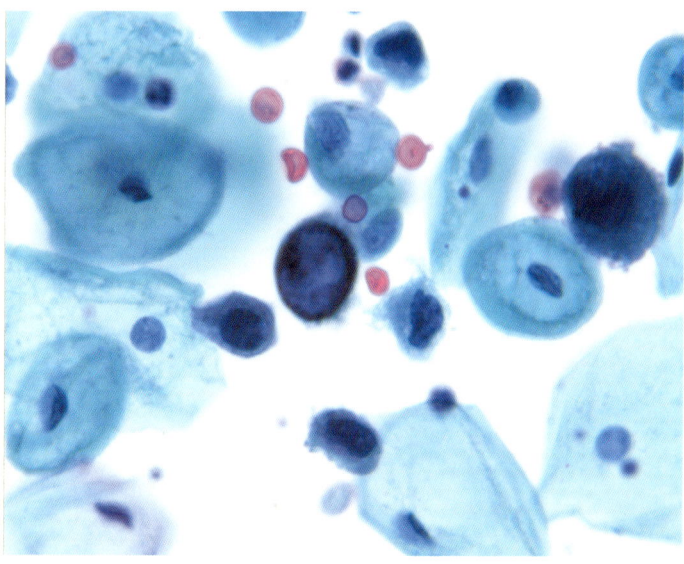

FIGURE 3.44. High Grade Urothelial Carcinoma with Polyoma Virus infected cells—voided urine: The central cell, greatly enlarged with very high NC ratio, is a prototypical polyoma virus infected cell with ground glass nucleus and margination of the chromatin. However, in the rest of the field are a variety of malignant cells from a high grade urothelial carcinoma. Compare the nucleus of the polyoma virus infected cell with the irregular nuclear shapes of the carcinoma cells. (600x)

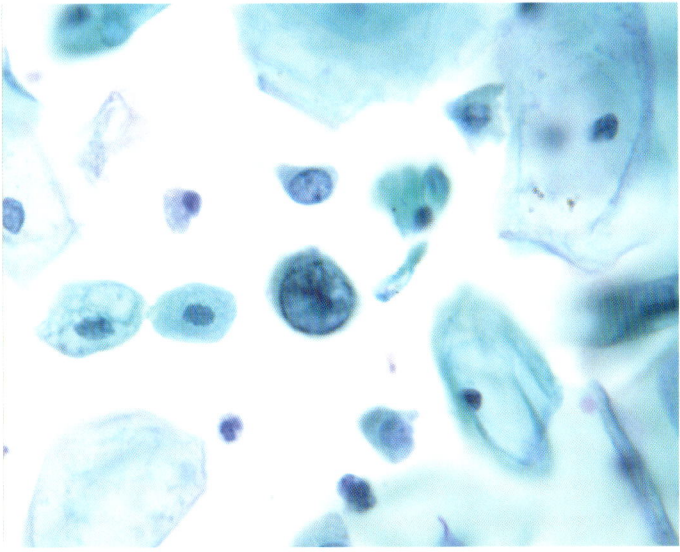

FIGURE 3.45. Polyoma Virus—voided urine: The ground glass nucleus is unusual by virtue of the light staining, marginated chromatin. The high NC ratio, round nuclear shape and generalized cellular enlargement is distinctly different from the smaller basal cell directly above the infected cell. Other squamous and urothelial cells surround the "decoy" cell. (600x)

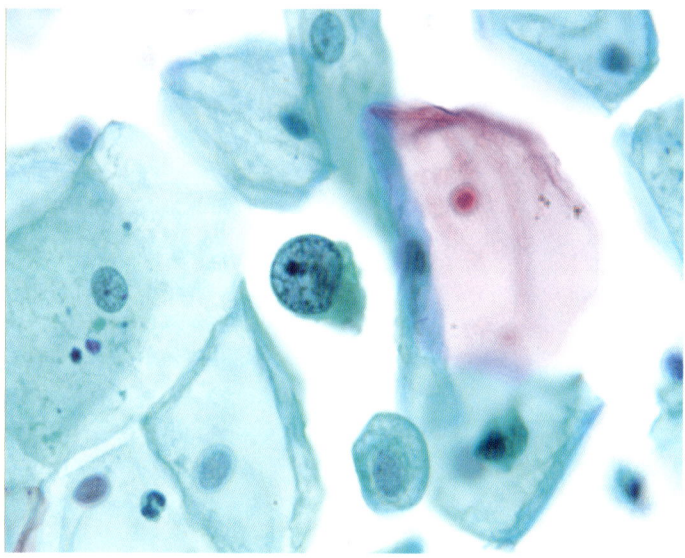

FIGURE 3.46. Polyoma Virus—voided urine: Features supporting polyoma virus infection are the enlarged cell, and round nucleus with a smooth border. This cell is not entirely characteristic as there is only partial ground glass dissolution of the nuclear chromatin leaving remnants of the nuclear matrix, and a prominent nucleolus. It may be a high grade urothelial carcinoma cell. Close follow-up of patients with such cellular changes is definitely warranted. (600x)

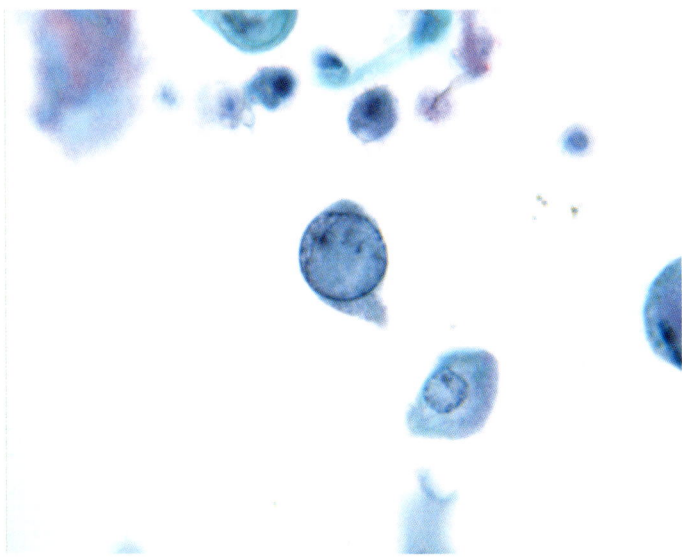

FIGURE 3.47. Polyoma Virus—voided urine: Although the classic polyoma virus infection renders the nucleus hyperchromatic, this particular cell is almost entirely cleared of nuclear chromatin. Compare the infected cell with the normal umbrella cell in the lower portion of the photograph. (600x)

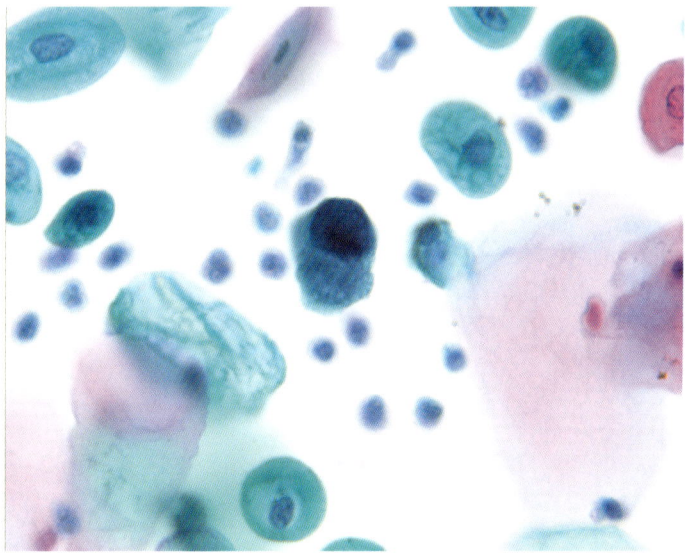

FIGURE 3.48. Polyoma Virus—voided urine: Although the nuclear chromatin changes are characteristic of polyoma virus, the irregular nuclear shape and the thin rim of cytoplasm around one edge of the nucleus is more suggestive of a high grade urothelial carcinoma. Careful follow-up of patients with such cells is warranted prompted by a cautionary note in the report. (600x)

Mimics of High Grade Urothelial Carcinoma 115

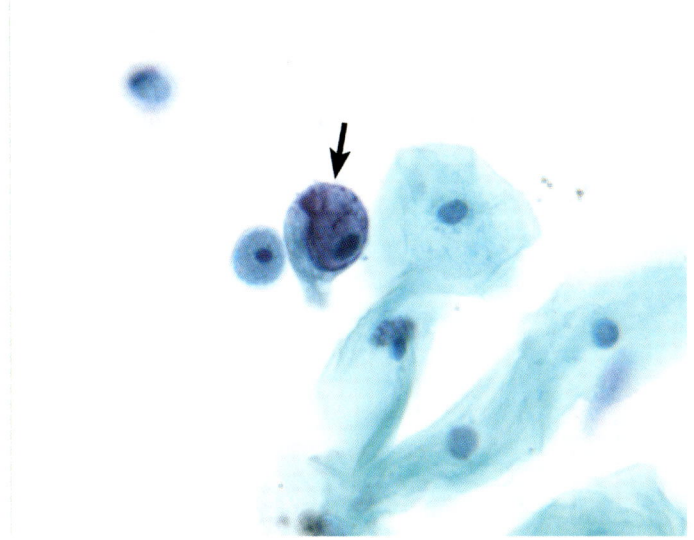

FIGURE 3.49. Polyoma Virus Infected High Grade Urothelial cell—voided urine: The infected cell (arrow) displays generalized cellular enlargement and ground glass areas within the nucleus, but the nuclear shape is not round, and a huge nucleolus is present. These latter two features suggest that the cell is malignant as well as infected with a virus. (600x)

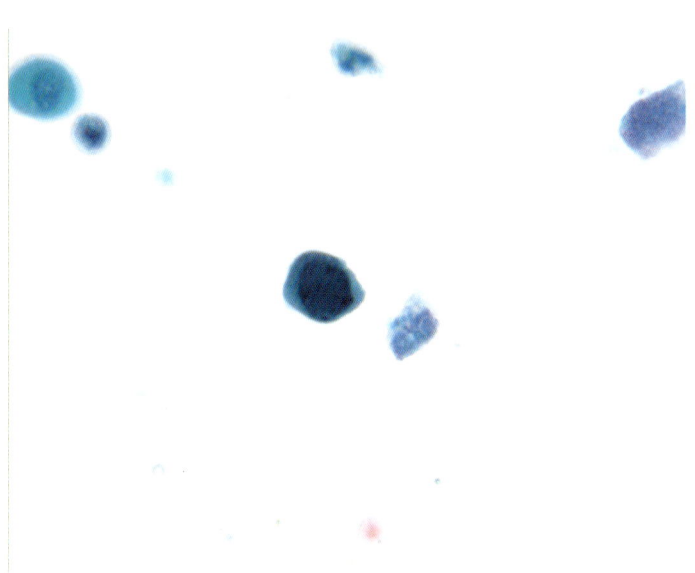

FIGURE 3.50. Polyoma Virus Infected Cell—voided urine: The cell is enlarged with high NC ratio and characteristic ground glass nuclear chromatin. Remnants of chromatin are located at the margin of the nucleus in clumps. (600x).

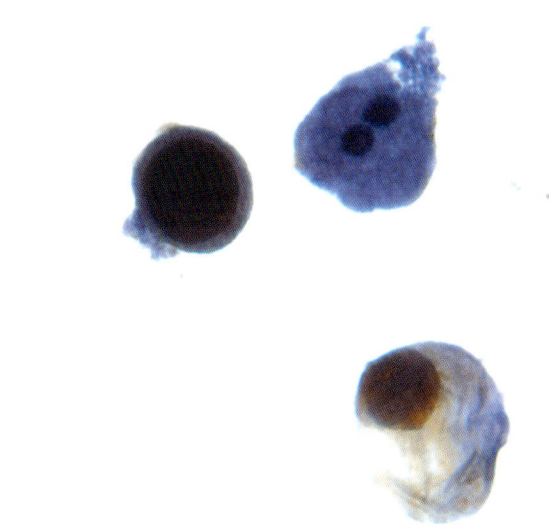

FIGURE 3.51. Polyoma virus infected cells stained with SV-40 immunochemical stain—voided urine: Numerous infected cells were recovered in the urine of a 46 year old male, suffering from chronic renal insufficiency secondary to Wegener's granulomatosis. He had been treated with steroids and cytoxan. Because of the number of abnormal cells, an SV-40 stain was used to exclude carcinoma in situ. The brown nuclear stain marks the infected enlarged cells; the binucleate umbrella cell is negative. The patient died 7 years later of his renal disease with no evidence on repeated urine samples of any urothelial neoplasm. (400x)

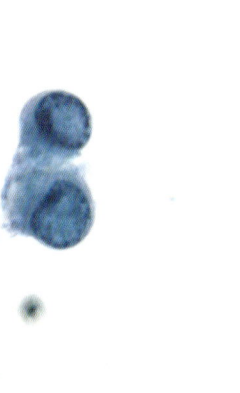

FIGURE 3.52. Polyoma Virus—voided urine: Infected cells are not always characterized by a dark nucleus. The ground glass dissolution of the nucleus, even when light in color, is characteristic of this virus, as are margination of the nuclear chromatin and smooth, round nuclear contours. However, high grade urothelial carcinoma cannot be entirely excluded when cells such as these are found in abundance in a sample. (600x)

Suggested Reading

Curry JL, Wojcik EM. The effects of the current World Health Organization/ International Society of Urologic Pathologists bladder neoplasm classification system on urine cytology results. Cancer Cytopathol 2002; 96:140–5.

Epstein JI, Amin MB, Reuter VR, Mostofi FK, and the Bladder Consensus Conference Committee: The World Health Organization/International Society of Urological Pathology consensus classification of urothelial (transitional cell) neoplasms of the urinary bladder. Am J of Surg Path 1998; 22:1435–1448.

Herawi M, Parwani AV, Epstein JI, Ali SZ. BK (Polyoma) virus-associated cellular changes in exfoliative urine and bladder biopsy samples: Is a cyto-histologic correlation possible? Acta Cytol 2004; 48:711.

Hughes JH, Raab SS, Cohen MB. The cytologic diagnosis of low grade transitional cell carcinoma. Am J Clin Pathol 2000; 114(Suppl 1): S59–S67.

Koss LG: Diagnostic Cytology and Its Histopathologic Bases, 4th edition. JB Lippincott, Philadelphia, 1992.

Koss LG: Diagnostic Cytology of the Urinary Tract. JB Lippincott, Philadelphia, 1995.

Koss LG: Tumors of the Urinary Bladder in Atlas of Tumor Pathology. HI Firminger, ed. Armed Forces Institute of Pathology, Washington, DC, 1975, pp. 24.

Lopez-Beltran A, Croghan GA, Croghan I, Matilla A, and Gaeta JF: Prognostic factors in bladder cancer: A pathologic, immunohistochemical, and DNA flow-cytometric study. Acta Cytol 1994; 38:109–114.

Mostofi FK, Sobin LH, Torloni H. Histological typing of urinary bladder tumors. In: International classification of tumors. No. 10 Geneva: World Health Organization, 1973. p. 15–17.

Murphy WM, Beckwith JB, Farrow GM: Tumors of the kidney, bladder, and related urinary structures in Atlas of Tumor Pathology, 3rd series, Fascicle 11. Armed Forces Institute of Pathology, Washington, DC, 1994, pp. 193–297.

Murphy WM, Crabtree WN, Jukkola AF, and Soloway MS: The diagnostic value of urine versus bladder washing in patients with bladder cancer. J Urol 1981; 126:320–322.

Murphy WM. Urinary Cytopathology. ASCP Press, Chicago, 2000.

Petersen RO: Urologic Pathology, 2nd edition. JB Lippincott, Philadelphia, 1992.

Raab SS, Lenel JC, Cohen MB. Low grade transitional cell carcinoma of the bladder. Cytologic diagnosis by key features as identified by logistic regression analysis. Cancer 1994; 74:1621–6.

Raab SS, Slagel DD, Jensen CS, Teague MW, Savell VH, Ozkutlu D, Lenel JC, Cohen MB. Low grade transitional cell carcinoma of the urinary bladder: application of select cytologic criteria to improve diagnostic accuracy. Mod Pathol 1996; 9:225–32.

Rosenthal DL: Urologic Cytology in Practical Cytopathology. RW Astarita, ed., Churchill Livingstone, New York, NY, 1990, pp. 303–336.

Witte D, Truong L, Ramzy I: Transitional Cell Carcinoma of the Renal Pelvis. Am J Clin Pathol 2002; 117:444–450.

Xin W, Raab SS, Michael CW. Low grade urothelial carcinoma: reappraisal of the cytologic criteria on ThinPrep. Diagn Cytopathol 2003; 29:125–9.

Zaman SS, Sack MJ, Ramchandani R, et al: Cytopathology of retrograde renal pelvis brush specimens: An analysis of 40 cases with emphasis on collecting duct carcinoma and low-intermediate grade transitional cell carcinoma. Diagn Cytopathol 1996; 15:312–321.

4
Special Circumstances

Ileal Loop or Neo-bladder

Surgical Considerations

A common surgical reconstruction transforms a loop of ileum into a "bladder" following cystectomy or ureteral diversion because of obstruction by inoperable neoplasm. The stoma exits through the skin into an external collecting bag. A neo-bladder replaces the surgically removed bladder with an isolated segment of large colon that is reanastamosed above the internal urethral sphincter; the ureters are spliced into an area approximating their original anatomic positions. Functional bladder reconstruction has enabled patients to accept cystectomy earlier in their disease process and has resulted in longer survival than if the bladder lesion became invasive, or the ureters were obstructed and destroyed the kidneys.

Cytologic Features

Samples from artificial bladders usually contain an abundance of enteric mucosal fragments, which often are degenerated and almost unrecognizable as glandular epithelium. Individual columnar cells more closely resemble degenerated small histiocytes than their true identity (Figs. 4.1–4.3). If the specimen is freshly prepared and the stain good, detecting tumor cells is not too difficult, as urothelial cells are substantially larger than degenerated enteric cells. If there is any suspicion of tumor, a repeat specimen is indicated.

The major problem occurs when neoplastic cells are found (Figs. 4.4–4.6). The ureters are difficult to cannulate through their new ostia, so that retrograde samples are not so easily obtained as when the ureters empty into the natural bladder. Therefore, the origin of tumor cells may not be determined by cystoscopic inspection. Imaging techniques may be the only way to localize the lesion.

Drug-Induced Cytologic Atypias

Drugs used for Treatment of Urothelial Neoplasms

Once the diagnosis of CIS is made, the clinician and patient are faced with the decision of cystectomy or conservative treatment. For most patients, cystectomy is a last resort. Three drugs have proven to be variably effective alternatives for the control of the high grade in situ lesions of the bladder. Bacille Calmette-Guerin (BCG), an attenuated bovine mycobacterium, Mitomycin, and Thiotepa may eradicate the neoplasm but result in an inflammatory reaction and urothelial atypia, and in the case of BCG, submucosal granulomas. The most success has been achieved with BCG and Mitomycin, with the former being less expensive.

Cytologic Criteria

When BCG is used as an intravesical agent, multinucleated histiocytes clustered with large monocytes and fibroblasts will indicate granulomatous reaction has occurred in the submucosa with erosion of the mucosa (Figs. 4.7–4.10). Occasionally, highly atypical urothelial cells will still be present soon after BCG therapy has ended (Figs. 4.11). The decision between reactive and persistent neoplastic cells presents a quandary for the cytologist. When in doubt—WAIT. A repeat specimen several months following the last treatment is prudent, and will clarify the predicament, for if the atypical cells persist, they are probably from residual cancer.

Drugs used for Treatment of Systemic Illness, not Specifically for Urothelial Disorders, which Produce Urothelial Atypia

The prototype of this problem is cyclophosphamide (cytoxan), a commonly used drug against lymphoproliferative neoplasms. The drug can produce an idiosyncratic reaction, characterized by hemorrhagic cystitis, as the drug is excreted in toxic quantities in the urine. There is no correlation between the cytologic atypia and the drug dosage, and although the changes may regress after discontinuing the drug, a few cases have reportedly progressed to invasive carcinoma.

Cytologic Criteria

The cytologic changes secondary to systemic pharmacologic agents are much like radiation reaction but are more pronounced (Figs. 4.12–4.16). There is variable cell enlargement with some preservation of the NC ratio, although the nuclear increase usually precedes the cytoplasmic changes. The enlarged nucleus may be eccentric, irregularly shaped, with marked hyperchromasia, coarse evenly distributed chromatin, presenting a "salt-and-pepper" appearance. The nucleolus may be enlarged and distorted in the very early changes. Later, nuclear pyknosis and karyorrhexis or a large and hyperchromatic nucleus with glassy chromatin will result. As in radiation change, the cytoplasm of urothelial cells is often vacuolated and sometimes contains particles of foreign material or neutrophils. Aberrant cytoplasmic shapes are frequently encountered. The most severe changes may "imitate urothelial carcinoma to perfection". (L.G. Koss)

In addition to cytoxan, busulfan has also been reported to produce severe cytologic atypias. As a practical rule, whenever a patient has a history of use of a cytotoxic agent, the urothelium may be a "target organ" and any cytologic changes must be viewed with skepticism. The need for complete clinical history is obvious.

Radiation-Induced Atypia

Many of the cytologic changes produced by external radiation, and described in samples from the female genital tract, are also seen in urinary samples from patients who may have received radiation to any of their pelvic organs. Benign urothelial cells that have been radiated display cellular enlargement with preservation of NC ratio, nuclear hyperchromasia, multinucleation and cytoplasmic vacuolization (Figs. 4.17–4.20). However, these changes can also be seen in urothelial cells that have not been radiated; these changes probably reflect generalized reactive phenomena. Loveless found in a well-controlled study that the most reliable change reflecting radiation effect on bladder epithelial cells was marked cellular enlargement. The distinction between radiation change in benign and malignant cells is based on generally accepted nuclear criteria of malignancy (Figs. 4.21, 4.22).

Lithiasis

The diagnostic treachery of urinary calculi is well established (see Table 6). Passage of a stone provokes not only blood and inflammatory cells, but also reactive changes including nuclear irregularities and hyperchromasia that can mimic carcinoma (Figs. 4.23). Usually, the cytologic changes will subside and virtually disappear once the calculus is passed. Therefore, if a history of stones is elicited, and the cytology is highly atypical, a few weeks' time will usually clarify the issue. If the atypia persists, a neoplasm must be excluded. Unfortunately, there is an increased occurrence of renal pelvic neoplasms coincident with renal pelvic calculi.

Ileal Loop 125

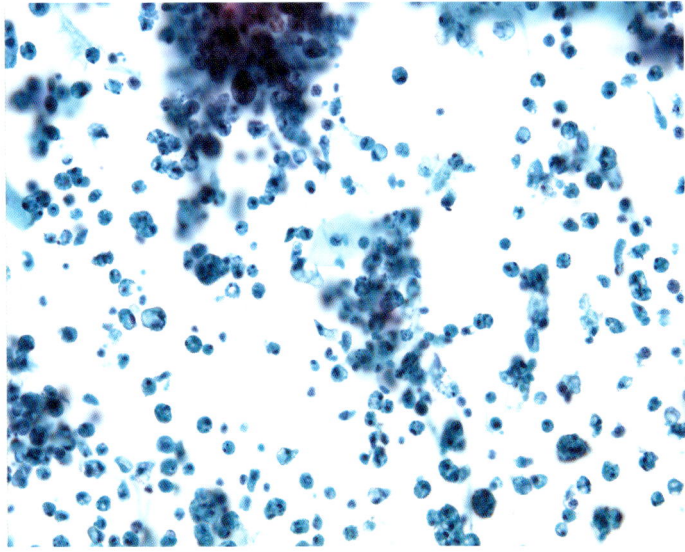

FIGURE 4.1. Enteric Cells—ileal loop: Specimens are usually highly cellular and consist primarily of degenerated enteric lining cells. Occasional clusters are seen but these cells are also degenerated and have small hyperchromatic nuclei. They should not be confused with a glandular lesion or neoplasm. (200x)

126 4. Special Circumstances

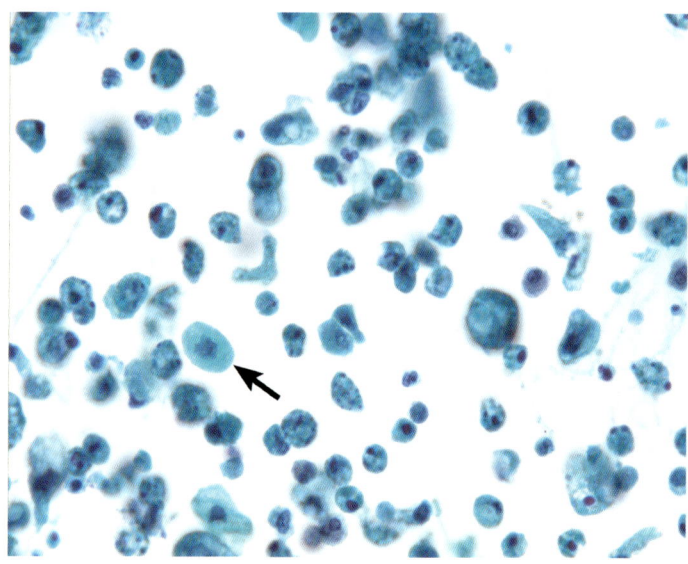

FIGURE 4.2. Enteric Cells—loop urine: Degenerated enteric epithelial cells usually are abundant and urothelial cells are rare (→) . (400x)

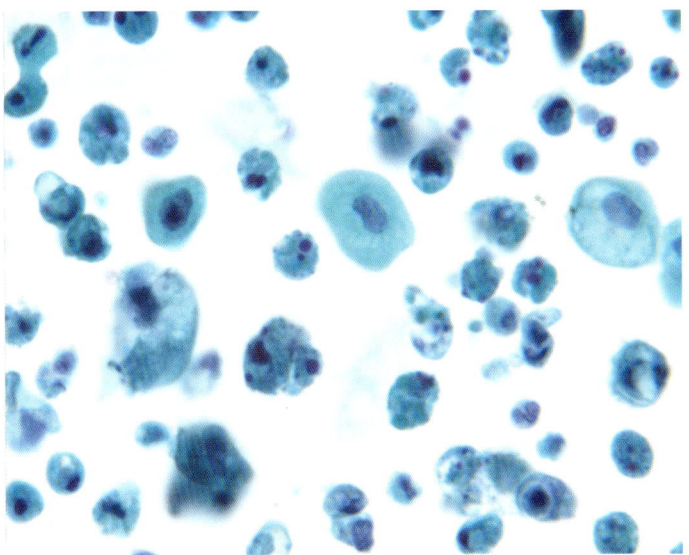

FIGURE 4.3. Normal Enteric and Urothelial Cells—ileal loop urine: The normal umbrella cells have well preserved nucleoli and abundant cytoplasm. They are also larger than the smaller degenerated enteric cells that resemble macrophages. (600x)

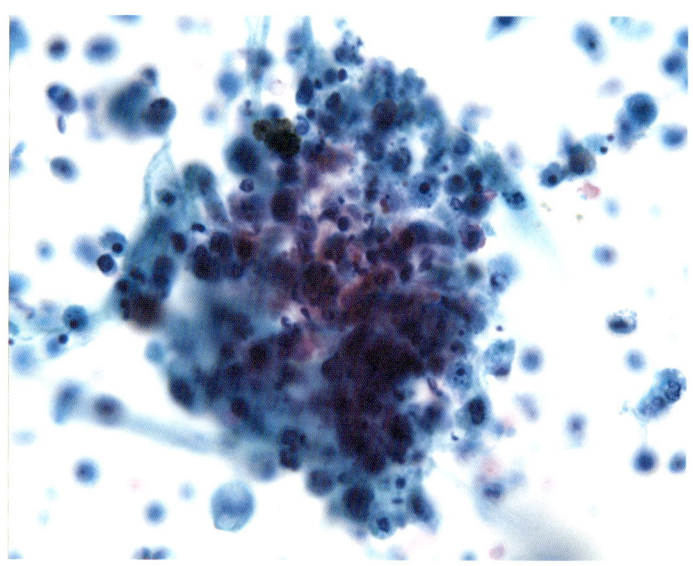

Figure 4.4. High Grade Urothelial Carcinoma—loop urine: Recurrent cancer presents with a variety of features, some of which are no more than cellular debris, suggesting tissue necrosis. Careful search for malignant urothelial cells is critical to render a definitive diagnosis of malignancy. (400x)

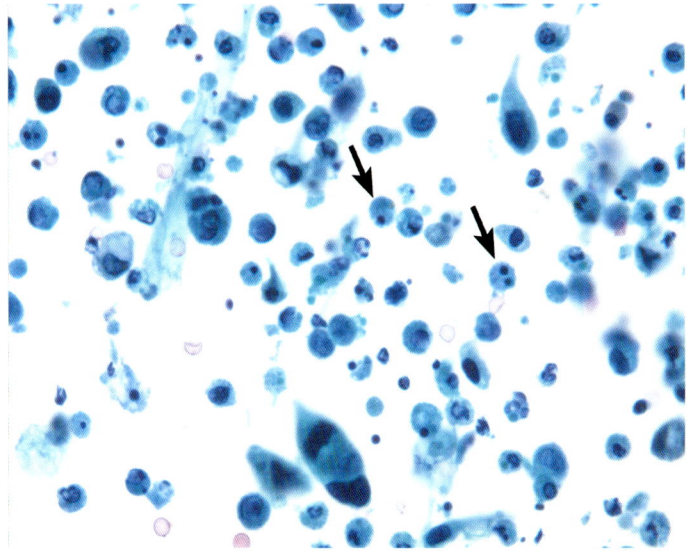

FIGURE 4.5. High Grade Urothelial Carcinoma—loop urine: Scattered high grade urothelial carcinoma cells are surrounded by smaller degenerated enteric epithelial cells (→) from an ileal loop following cystectomy. Most of the cancer cells are much larger than the enteric cells. There are some tumor cells that are small but their high NC ratios and nuclear features are evidence of their malignancy. (400x)

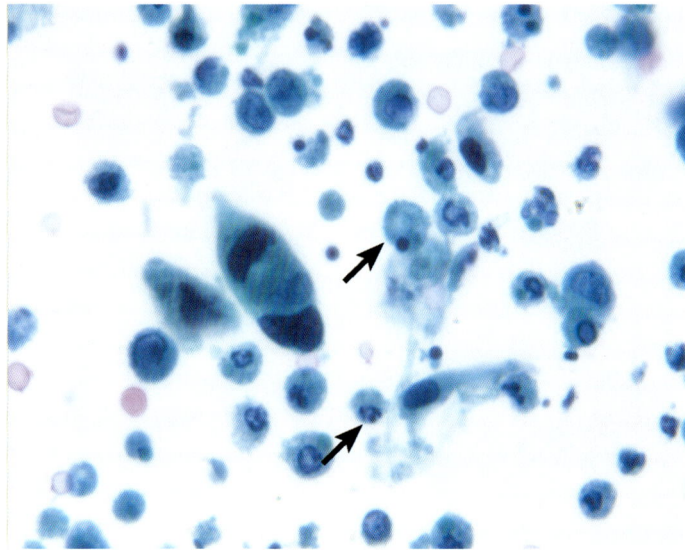

FIGURE 4.6. High Grade Urothelial Carcinoma—loop urine: Malignant cells of varying sizes, but all with enlarged nuclei and high NC ratios, are contrasted with smaller degenerated enteric epithelial cells (→). (600x)

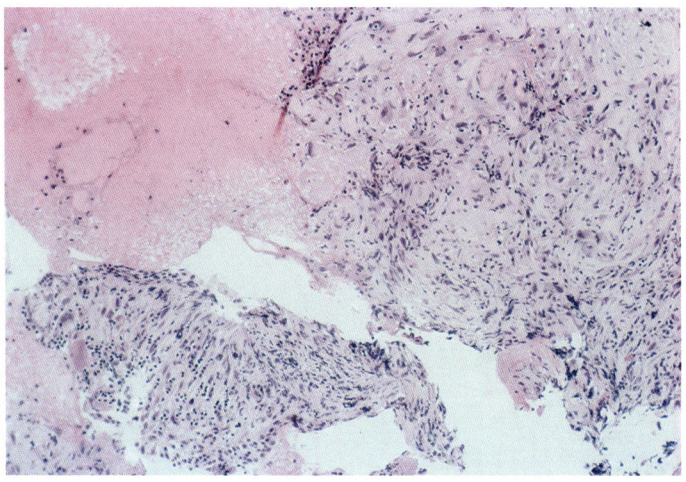

FIGURE 4.7. BCG Therapy—bladder biopsy: Conservative therapy for in situ bladder cancer usually includes a series of BCG instillations. The almost immediate cellular reaction is denudation of the mucosa and development of submucosal granulomas. (H&E, 200x)

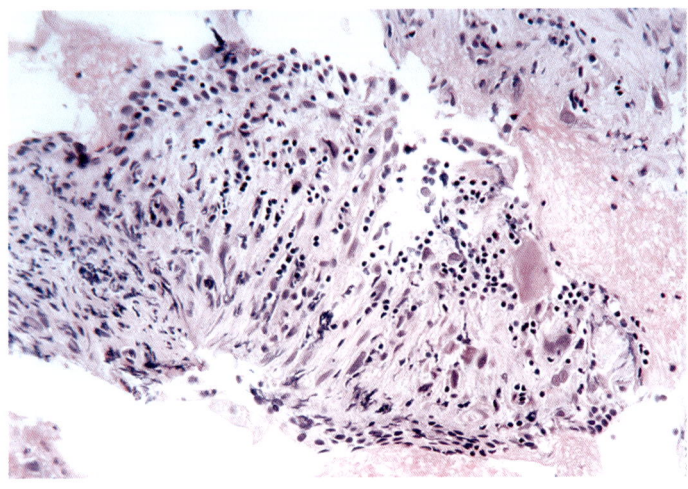

FIGURE 4.8. BCG Therapy—bladder biopsy: A closer look at the non-caseating granulomas confirms the assortment of lymphocytes, fibroblasts and macrophages. (H&E, 400x)

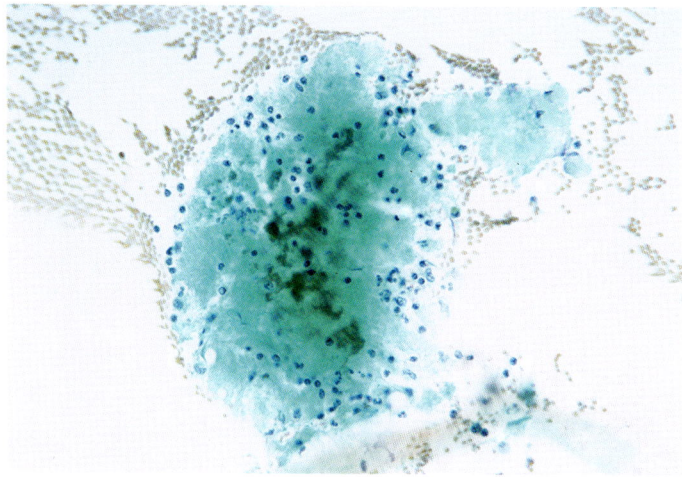

FIGURE 4.9. BCG Therapy—bladder washing: Dense coagulum is a common finding following BCG instillations, and reflects the leaking of serum through the denuded urothelium. (200x)

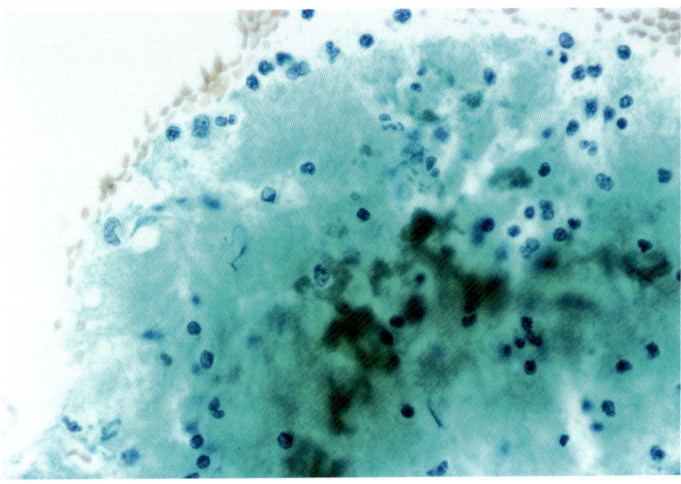

FIGURE 4.10. BCG Therapy—bladder washing: Closer examination of the coagulum discloses entrapped lymphocytes. (400x)

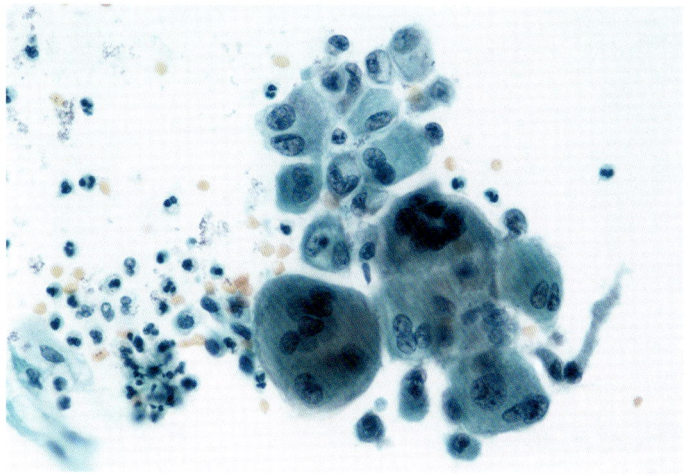

FIGURE 4.11. BCG Therapy—bladder washing: Occasional multinucleated histocytes are recovered in a sample, reflecting the granulomatous process. They should not be confused with residual tumor cells that will have larger and more hyperchromatic nuclei, and higher NC ratios. (400x)

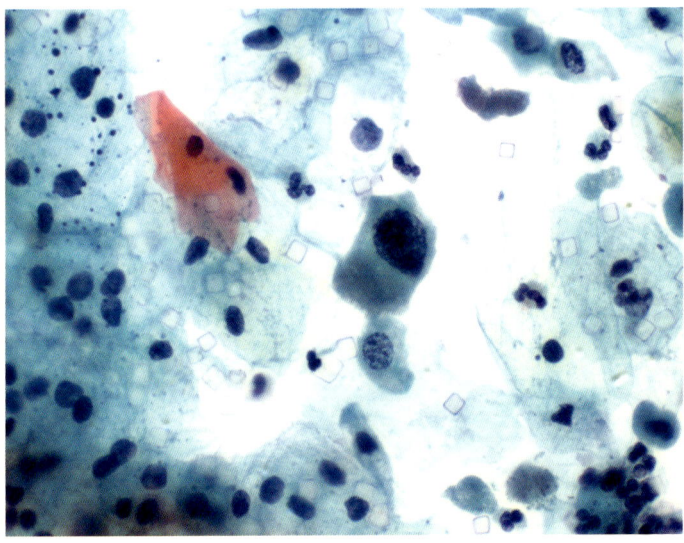

FIGURE 4.12. Chemotherapy Effect—bladder washing: In this bladder washing specimen, a large atypical cell is seen in the center of the field. The cell has an enlarged nucleus with marked hyperchromasia. However, the nuclear to cytoplasmic ratio is not increased and the cytoplasm has a reparative appearance. A background of acute inflammation and benign squamous and urothelial cells is seen. This cell is representative of chemotherapy effect. (600x)

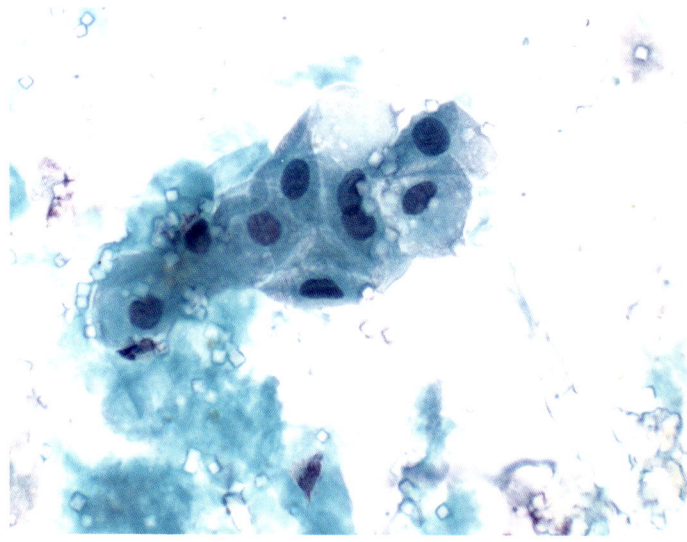

FIGURE 4.13. Chemotherapy Effect—bladder washing: A cluster of atypical urothelial cells is observed. These cells have a moderate amount of cytoplasm although the nuclei are slightly atypical and a binucleated cell is seen. The nuclei are round to oval. Crystals are seen in the background. This patient has a history of uterine cancer and systemic chemotherapy. (600x)

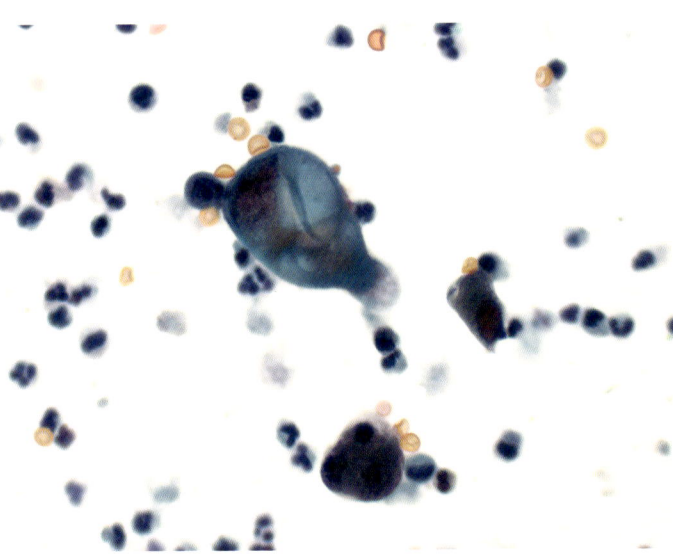

FIGURE 4.14. Chemotherapy Effect—catheterized urine: Acute inflammatory cells are seen with degenerated atypical urothelial cells in this patient with a history of chemotherapy. In the center field is a large binucleated urothelial cell that contains abundant cytoplasm and prominent cytoplasmic vacuoles, although the nuclear chromatin is hyperchromatic and the nuclear membranes are irregular. The low nuclear to cytoplasmic ratio and the abundant cytoplasm indicate that the findings are most likely that of chemotherapy effect. (600x)

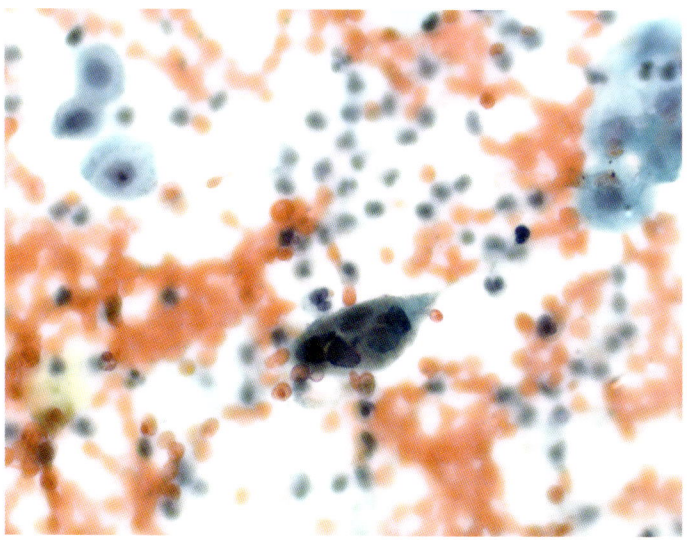

FIGURE 4.15. Chemotherapy Effect—bladder washing: A cluster of atypical hyperchromatic urothelial cells is seen in this patient who has a history of chemotherapy. A background of acute inflammation and benign urothelial cells is seen. The atypical cells exhibit irregular nuclear membranes although the nuclei are degenerated. (600x)

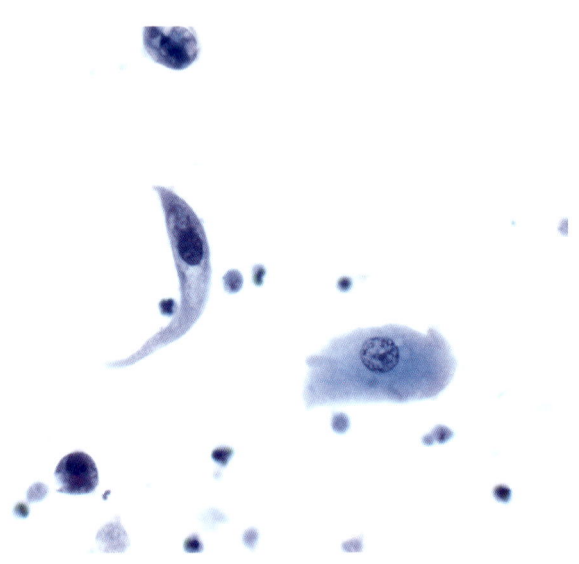

FIGURE 4.16. Chemotherapy Effect—bladder washing: Atypical urothelial cells are admixed with acute inflammation and degenerated and benign urothelial cells. In the center of the field is a cell with abundant cytoplasm and a degenerated small hyperchromatic nucleus. Cytoplasmic tails may be seen in chemotherapy effect. (600x)

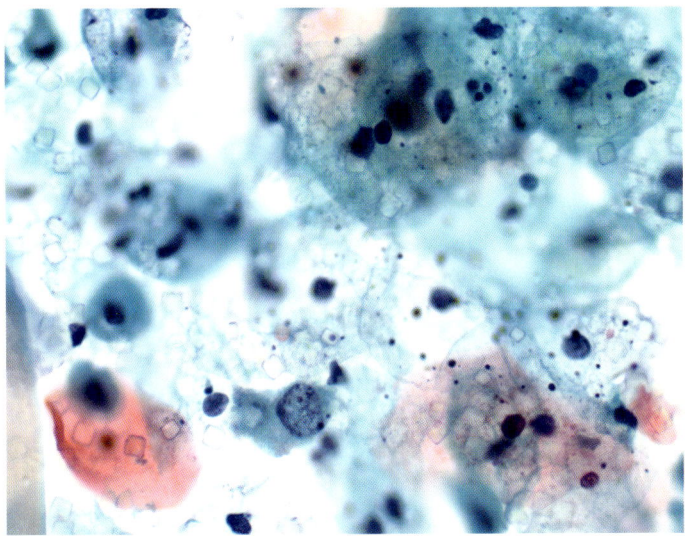

FIGURE 4.17. Radiation Effect—bladder washing: An atypical urothelial cell is seen in the bottom center field. The cell has an enlarged nucleus and a moderate amount of basophilic cytoplasm. The nucleus has a degenerated quality, and in the background, degenerated debris, crystals and benign squamous cells are seen. (600x)

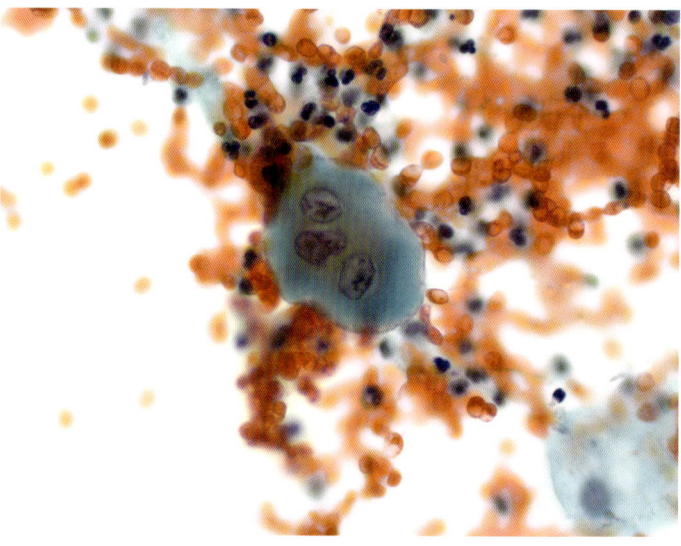

FIGURE 4.18. Radiation Effect—bladder washing: A multinucleated atypical urothelial cell is admixed with abundant blood, debris, and neutrophils. Superficial urothelial cells may exhibit significant radiation effect, including nuclear hyperchromasia, nuclear membrane irregularities, and nuclear membrane thickening. (600x)

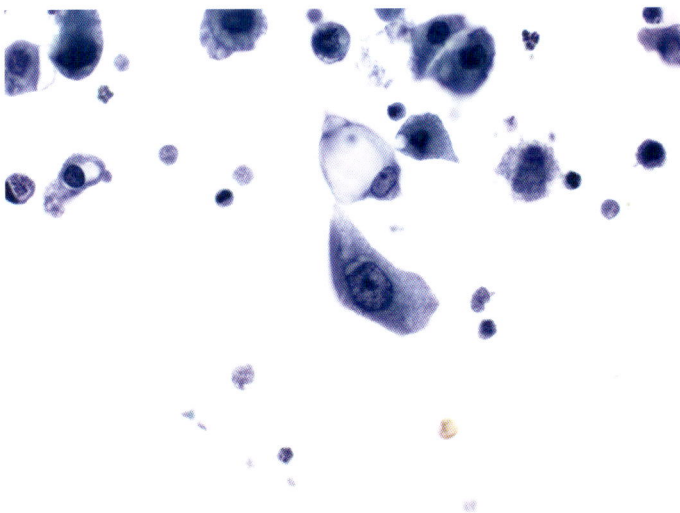

FIGURE 4.19. Radiation Effect—bladder washing: Atypical, degenerated urothelial cells are seen. These atypical cells exhibit a slightly increased nuclear to cytoplasmic ratio and nuclear membrane irregularities. The nuclei are slightly hyperchromatic. The cytoplasm exhibits vacuolization and degeneration, features typical of radiation effect. (600x)

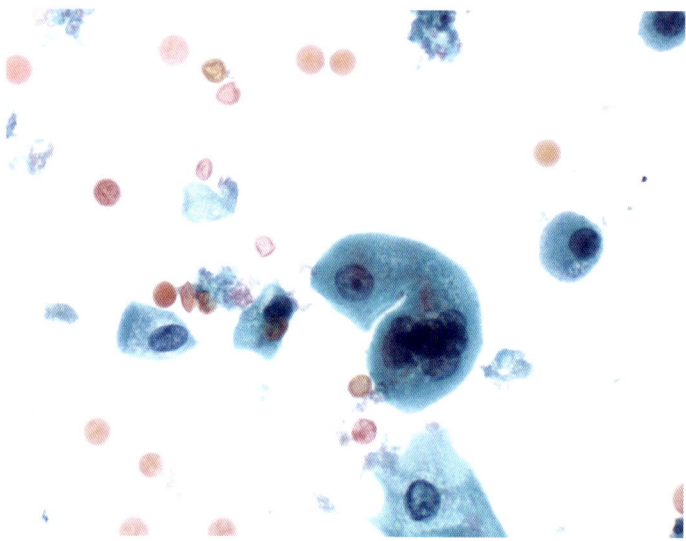

FIGURE 4.20. Radiation Effect—bladder washing: A multinucleated urothelial cell is seen in this patient who has undergone radiation treatment. The cells show multiple overlapping nuclei, as well as an eccentrically placed nucleus in the same cell. The nuclei have small nucleoli. (600x)

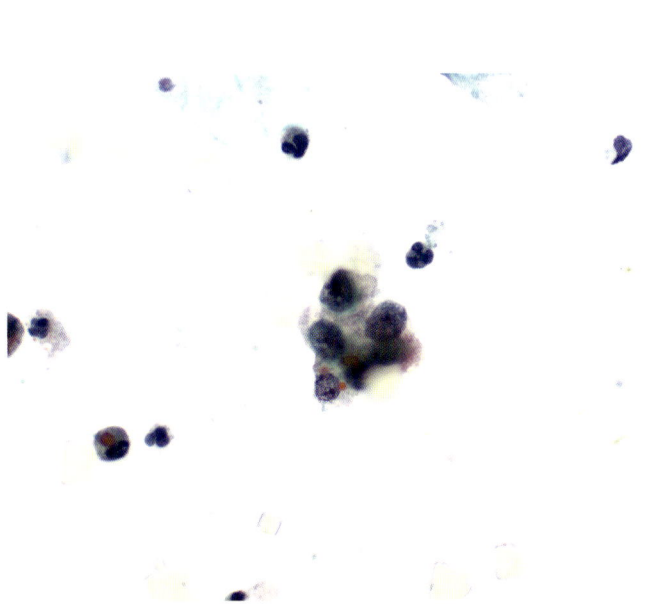

FIGURE 4.21. Radiation Effect—voided urine: Atypical urothelial cells are admixed with acute inflammatory cells and crystals. The atypical cells show high nuclear to cytoplasmic ratios, although extensive nuclear and cytoplasmic degeneration is seen. Prominent nucleoli also are observed. Although this case may be diagnosed as atypical, the follow-up indicated that this patient had radiation therapy and biopsies did not show an urothelial carcinoma. (600x)

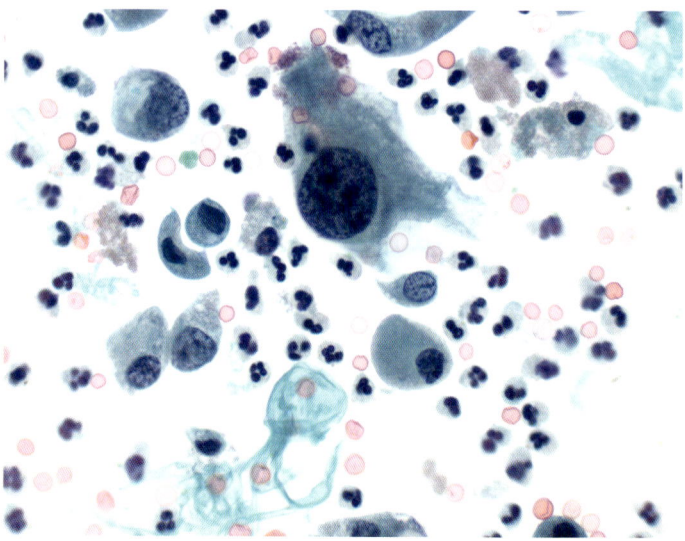

FIGURE 4.22. High Grade Urothelial Carcinoma and Radiation Effect—catheterized urine: Malignant urothelial cells are admixed with acute inflammatory cells and extensive degeneration in this patient who has a history of radiation. The largest cell is seen in the center and the nucleus is huge and hyperchromatic although the cell exhibits a moderate amount of cytoplasm and cytoplasmic tails that may be seen in either radiation or chemotherapy effect. However, the other cells that are observed also most likely represent malignant urothelial cells. These cells have lower nuclear to cytoplasmic ratios although the nuclei are hyperchromatic and irregular in shape. (600x)

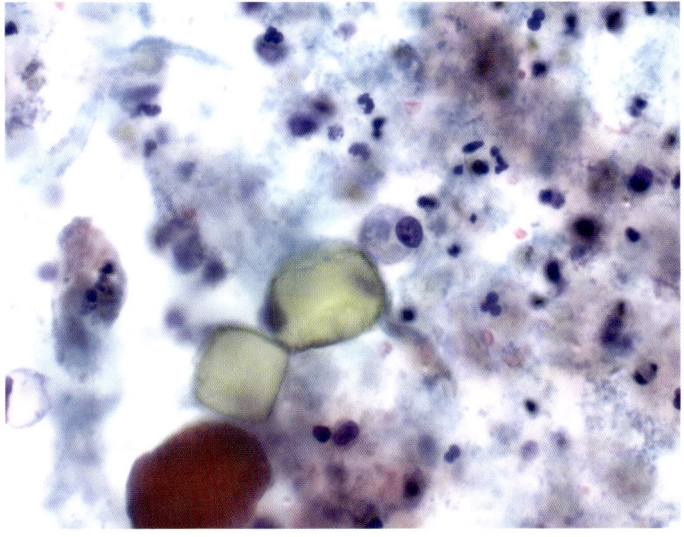

FIGURE 4.23. Lithiasis—voided urine: In lithiasis specimens, there often is abundant acute inflammation, debris and crystals. In this case, only rare intact urothelial cells are present admixed with debris. (600x)

Suggested Reading

Koss LG: Diagnostic Cytology and Its Histopathologic Bases, 4th edition. JB Lippincott, Philadelphia, 1992.

Koss LG: Diagnostic Cytology of the Urinary Tract. JB Lippincott, Philadelphia, 1995.

Rosenthal DL: Urologic Cytology in Practical Cytopathology. RW Astarita, ed., Churchill Livingstone, New York, NY, 1990, pp. 303–336.

5
Unusual Lesions

Size limits of this volume preclude a complete description of the various uncommon lesions of the urinary tract. The interested reader is referred to the classic texts of Koss, and other books relative to urinary cytology.

Lesions Arising in the Bladder

Squamous carcinoma and adenocarcinoma are infrequent cancers in the bladder, but have the same characteristics as those lesions elsewhere in the body (Figs. 5.1–5.3). The microscopist should resist the temptation to call a urothelial lesion "squamous" or "glandular" when areas of squamous or glandular metaplasia are encountered in an otherwise clear-cut urothelial carcinoma. The treatment is much more aggressive for the non-urothelial lesions.

Lesions Arising in the Kidney

Renal cell carcinoma (RCC) rarely sheds into the urine, and then only at a late stage, so that urinary cytology is not an appropriate screening test for that lesion. While the cells of renal cell carcinoma are classically described as having very prominent nucleoli, they are not always so. Deceptively small and inconspicuous nucleoli are often present in cells of well-differentiated RCC and can be very misleading. Clinical setting and suspicion are of great assistance in reaching an accurate diagnosis. Fine needle aspiration is the preferred approach to lesions of the renal parenchyma. However, cells from cystic renal cell carcinoma can mimic macrophages expected in a benign renal cyst. Ploidy studies and immunochemistry can be very helpful when sufficient material is aspirated.

Metastases to the Urinary Tract

Metastatic lesions to the urinary bladder and into ureters must be considered when history is consistent or when an unexpected cell population is found. Rectum, uterus, vagina, and prostate are contiguous and may be sources of direct spread (Figs. 5.4–5.6). Voided urines from women with occult gynecologic lesions may contain diagnostic cells in the urine (Figs. 5.7–5.11). Therefore, any woman presenting with "hematuria" should be catheterized to avoid vaginal contamination and to localize the source of bleeding. Drop metastases into the pouch of Douglas, or onto the dome of the bladder occur from distant sites. A complete and accurate history obviously is necessary to include such lesions in the differential diagnosis (Tables 8 and 9).

TABLE 8. Differential Diagnosis of Glandular Cells in Urine

Normal glandular epithelium
Cystitis Cystica
Gynecologic
   -Menstrual endometrium
   -Endometriosis
   -Normal endocervical cells
   -Malignancies
Retrograde ejaculation
Prostate, benign and malignant
Adenocarcinoma
   -Bladder
   -Metastatic to the bladder

TABLE 9. Differential Diagnosis of Squamous Cells in Urine

Normal squamous epithelium
Squamous metaplasia (usually trigonal)
    -Post inflammation
    -Post therapy
Vaginal contamination (voided urine)
Well-differentiated squamous carcinoma
Skin

5. Unusual Lesions

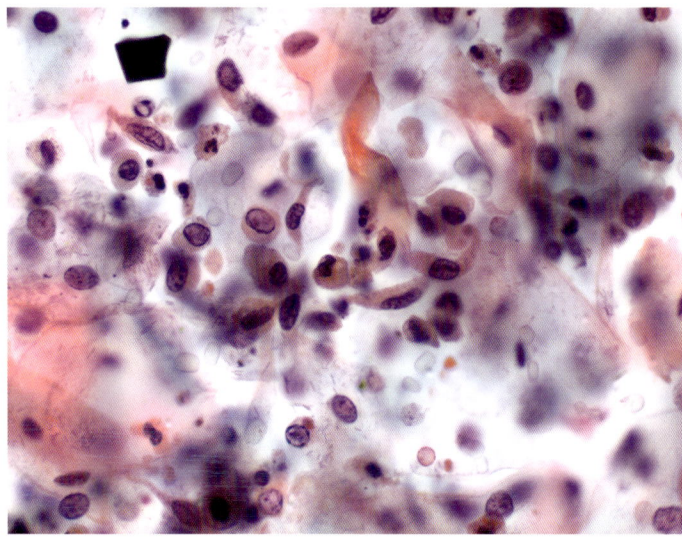

FIGURE 5.1. Squamous Carcinoma—bladder washing: Malignant squamous cells are admixed with degenerated debris, crystals, acute inflammation and blood. The malignant cells have an elongated appearance, and the cytoplasm is keratinized. (600x)

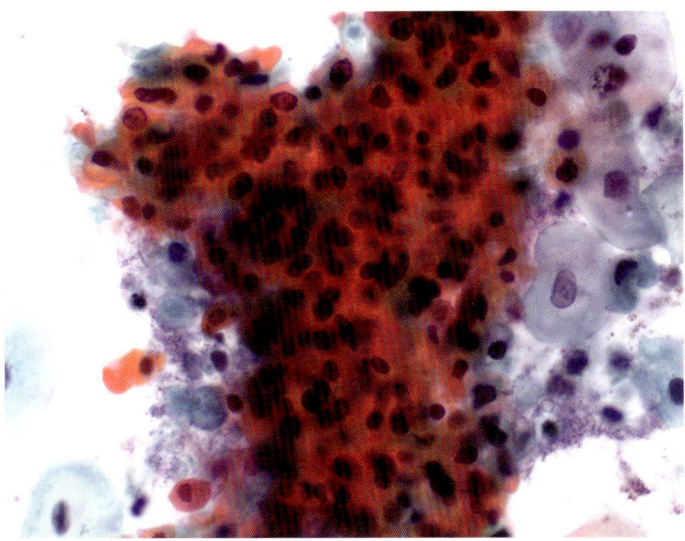

FIGURE 5.2. Squamous Carcinoma—bladder washing: In some squamous cell carcinomas, the cells have a very bland appearance, and only slight nuclear enlargement and mild nuclear hyperchromasia are evident. In some cases the cells exhibit dysplastic features rather than features of an invasive squamous cell carcinoma. (600x)

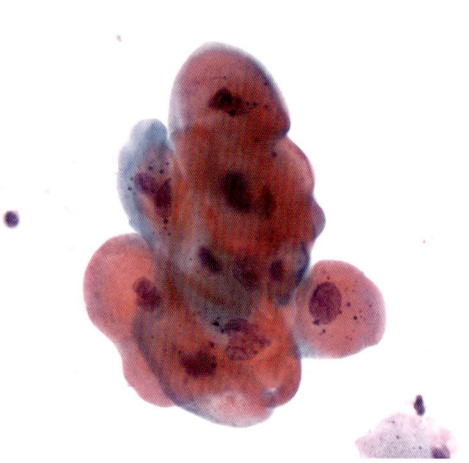

FIGURE 5.3. Squamous Carcinoma—bladder washing: The malignant cells exhibit only a slightly increased nuclear to cytoplasmic ratio. The cells in this case show mild nuclear hyperchromasia and nuclear membrane irregularities. (600x)

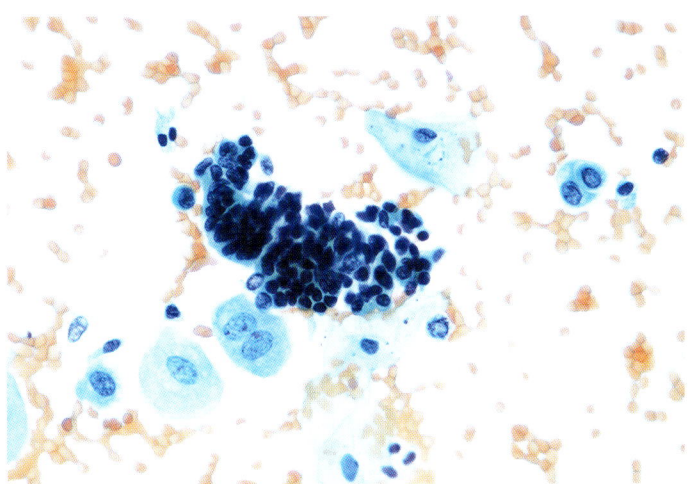

FIGURE 5.4. Endometriosis—ureteral washing: Unexpected cells warrant careful gathering of clinical information. This sample was obtained from the ureter of a 36 year old woman who suffered from intermittent obstruction of her ureter, coincident with her menstrual cycles. (400x)

156   5. Unusual Lesions

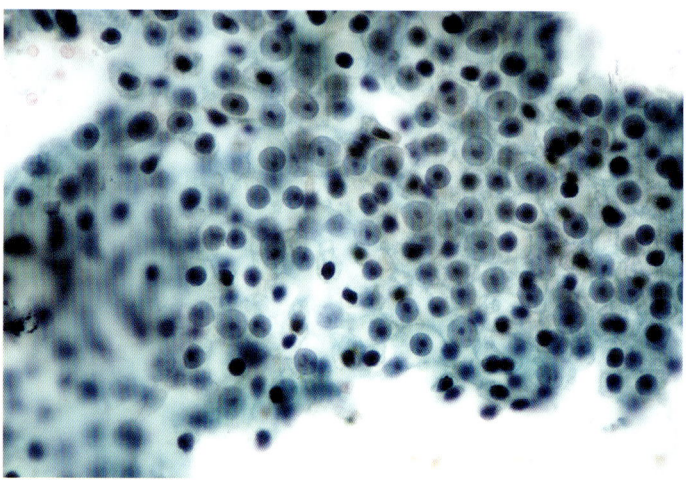

FIGURE 5.5. Carcinoma of the Prostatic Duct—urethral brush: Bladder outlet obstruction prompted brushing of the trigone area of an older gentleman. Sheets of uniformly large cells with dramatically round and central nuclei were confusing, as they were obviously malignant and yet were not consistent with a urothelial lesion. (400x)

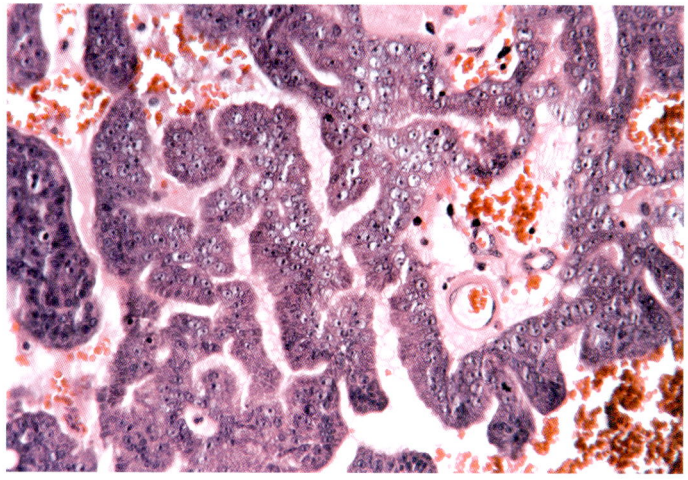

FIGURE 5.6. Carcinoma of the Prostatic Duct—urethral biopsy: The cytologic features in the biopsy are identical to those in the brushing of the lesion, rendering it a high grade classification. (H&E, 400x)

158   5. Unusual Lesions

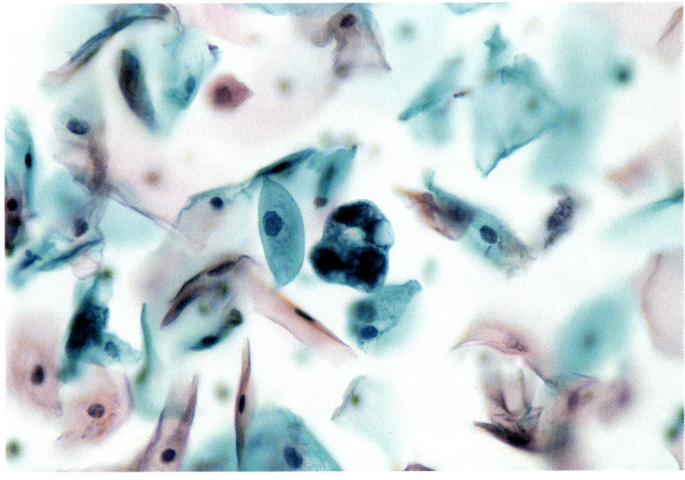

FIGURE 5.7. Carcinoma of the ovary—voided urine: In a urine contaminated with vaginal epithelial cells, rare groups of glandular cells were recovered. Although they could have arisen from the uterus, their large size and absence of accompanying blood urged us to get additional history. (600x)

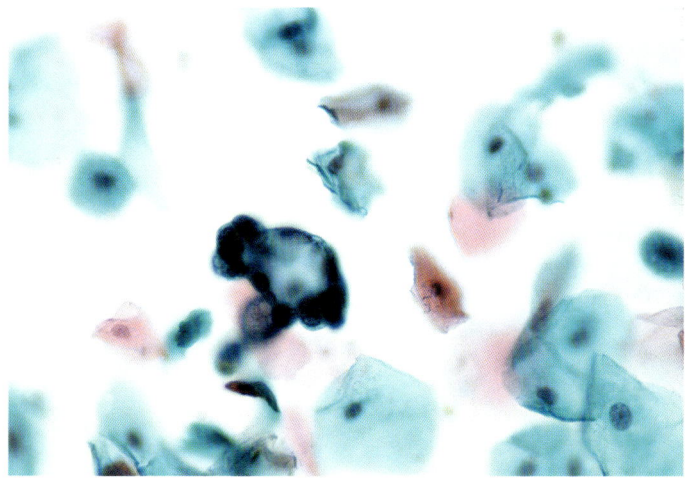

FIGURE 5.8. Carcinoma of the ovary—voided urine: Another glandular group from the same sample as 5.7. Their 3-dimensional quality is evidenced by the different focal plane of the cells in the background. (600x)

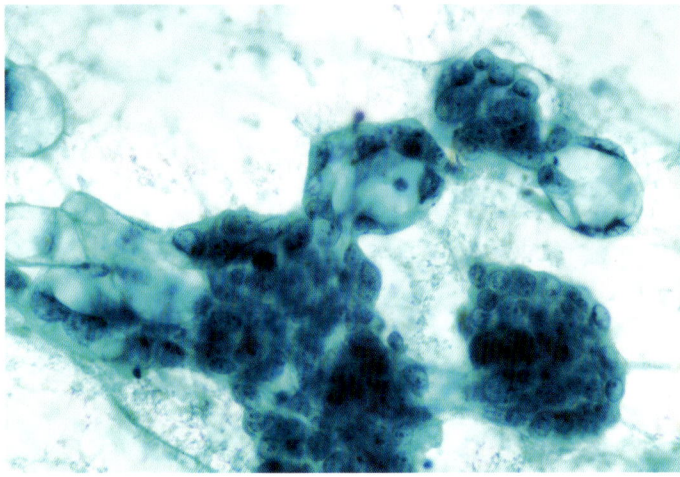

FIGURE 5.9. Carcinoma of the ovary—cervical smear: Several weeks prior to the patient's urine collection (Figs. 5.7, 5.8), a Pap test was interpreted as "Atypical glandular cells, favor a neoplasm". These groups of cells appear too large to be from either the cervix or uterus, but are clearly neoplastic and of glandular origin. (600x)

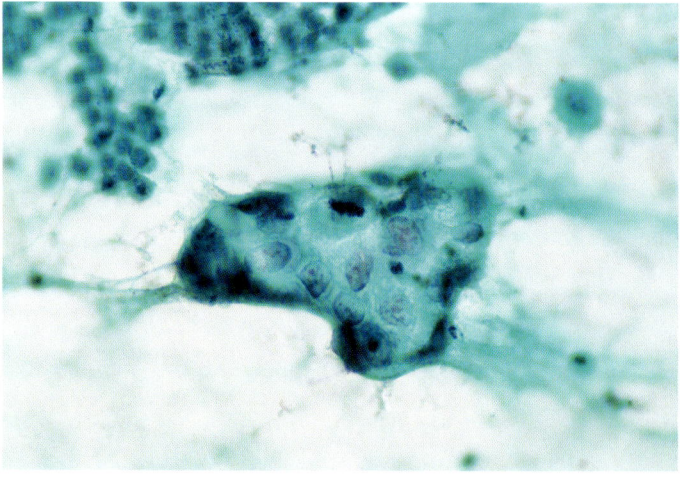

FIGURE 5.10. Carcinoma of the ovary—cervical smear: Another field of view from the Pap test pictured in Figure 5.9. (600x)

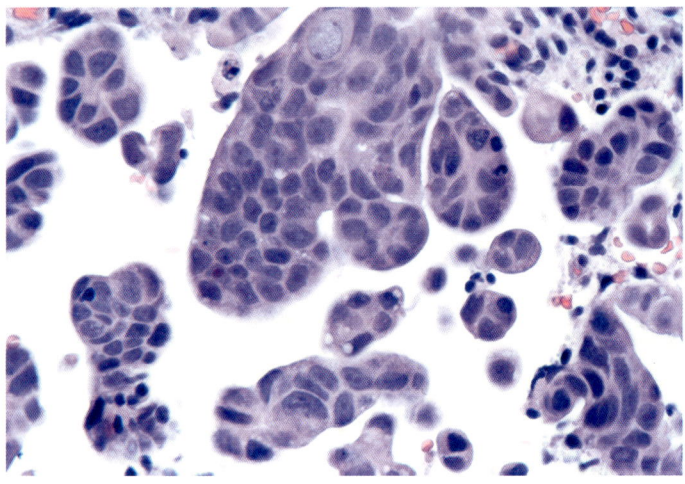

FIGURE 5.11. Carcinoma of the ovary—resection of tumor: Cellular features of this patient's ovarian carcinoma reveals its high grade. Immunohistochemical phenotyping placed the tumor in a serous category, but its cytologic features include prominent vacuolization. (H&E, 400x)

Suggested Reading

Koss LG: Diagnostic Cytology and Its Histopathologic Bases, 4th edition. JB Lippincott, Philadelphia, 1992.

Koss LG: Diagnostic Cytology of the Urinary Tract. JB Lippincott, Philadelphia, 1995.

Murphy WM, Crabtree WN, Jukkola AF, and Soloway MS: The diagnostic value of urine versus bladder washing in patients with bladder cancer. J Urol 1981; 126:320–322.

Rosenthal DL: Urologic Cytology in Practical Cytopathology. RW Astarita, ed., Churchill Livingstone, New York, NY, 1990, pp. 303–336.

Wiener HG, Vooijs GP, and van't Hof-Grootenboer B: Accuracy of urinary cytology in the diagnosis of primary and recurrent bladder cancer. Acta Cytol 1993; 37(2): 163–169.

6
Performance Characteristics of Urinary Cytology

Correlation Between Cytology and Histology

Most organ systems from which specimens are examined by both cytology and histology will provide immediate correlation between the cytologic and histologic diagnoses if the samples are obtained correctly. The urinary tract, on the contrary, is often a source of much frustration for both the clinician and the pathologist. In our experience, and that of others, a year or more may elapse between the initial "positive" cytologic diagnosis indicating a urothelial neoplasm and the confirming biopsy. In the interim, multiple negative biopsies may be obtained before the illusive source of the malignant cells is found. After a few such experiences shared by the confused urologist and initially embarrassed pathologist, the urologist may well begin treatment of such a patient based on positive cytologic findings, even without a confirming tissue diagnosis.

Even more serious is the occasion in which there is cytologic evidence of an invasive lesion suggested by high grade neoplastic cells, blood, and necrotic debris, and a tissue biopsy that will not verify the diagnosis. Then, the ureters and upper tract should be investigated, and if no radiologic evidence is found, random biopsies may be indicated. The phenomenon of "denudation" has been addressed in chapter 3, and should be considered when epithelium is partially or completely absent from a cup biopsy.

Histologic and cytologic samples that are obtained at the same time or within temporal proximity should be examined together so that the source of any cellular atypia can be determined. If the cytologic diagnosis is not histologically verified, such a comment should be included in the biopsy report so that the urologist knows that further search must be undertaken. As indicated above, there may be considerable time between the discovery of significantly atypical cells in a urine sample and the final verifying biopsy. Additionally, a biopsy from the bladder may reveal a low grade lesion, while the cytology may suggest that a significantly higher grade lesion is present. Either a focus of carcinoma in situ of the bladder must be sought, or a higher grade lesion within the upper tracts must be located. Therefore, an identical match between cytology and histology should be considered a "correlation". If even a moderate discrepancy is noted, diagnoses should be considered discordant.

Diagnostic Yield of Urinary Cytology

Dependance of Accuracy on Grade of Tumors

Perhaps the most well summarized evaluation of the usefulness of urinary cytology in the detection of tumors of the urinary tract has been made by Farrow. His data from 10,000 patients emphasize the low yield for the low grade papillary lesions, in contrast to the excellent diagnostic level for the high grade lesions. However, it should be noted that despite the low accuracy for low grade lesions these lesions still may be detected in specific scenarios. Farrow further emphasizes the importance of combining cystoscopic findings with cytologic changes to arrive at the optimum diagnosis for a given patient. Results from Farrow's study can be summarized as follows:

1. <u>Size of tumor</u>: Total surface area of a bladder tumor or tumors correlates with cytologic result, i.e., the greater the surface area, the more likely the diagnosis is to be "positive".
2. <u>Configuration of tumor</u>: Sessile (implying invasion) tumors, and carcinomas in situ are more readily diagnosed than the papillary tumors, i.e., 73% "positive" for CIS or sessile vs. 37% "positive" for papillary lesions.

3. <u>Grade of tumor</u>: Out of 634 histologically confirmed tumors:
   Grade   I (98 pts)   —   22% "positive" results
              II (291 pts) —   62% "positive" results
              III (215 pts) —   84% "positive" results
              IV (30 pts) —   83% "positive" results
4. <u>Negative cystoscopy vs. positive or suspicious cytology</u>: In patients with initially negative cystoscopic exams and negative biopsies, but with significant cytologic atypia, the great majority was subsequently proven to have cancer somewhere in the urinary tract. The need for long-term follow-up of abnormal urinary cytologies is underscored.
5. <u>Overall reliability of urinary cytology for detection of bladder cancer</u>:
   Sensitivity, overall   −66.6% (true positive)
   Specificity, overall   −95.4% (true negative)

Wiener et al. collected data from 263 patients with new and recurrent bladder "disorders". Using the results of 2213 cytologic examinations they conclude that diagnostic accuracy is directly related to histologic grade of the tumor, with the higher the grade the higher the correlation. Treatment of tumors degrades the accuracy of follow-up specimens. The most recent analysis of the utility of urinary cytology by Bastacky et al. reinforces experience: high correlation with high grade lesions, discouraging results with low grade neoplasms. While their overall results (Table 10) are essentially identical to those of Farrow, the variation among the three laboratories casts a shadow of unreliability on urinary tract cytology.

TABLE 10. Sensitivity, Specificity, Negative (NPV) and Positive Predictive Values (PPV)

	Overall %	Lab # 1%	Lab # 2%	Lab # 3%
Sensitivity	64	47	85	66
Specificity	95	98	74	98
PPV	75	81	56	88
NPV	92	91	93	94
Accuracy	89	90	77	96

Suggested Reading

Badalament RA: Editorial: Is the role of cystoscopy in the detection of bladder cancer really declining? J Urol 1998; 159:399–400.

Bastacky S, Ibrahim S, Wilczynski SP, Murphy WM: The accuracy of urinary cytology in daily practice. Cancer Cytopathol 1999; 87:118–128.

Farrow GM: Urine Cytology of Transitional Cell Carcinoma: Diagnostic Efficacy in Compendium on Diagnostic Cytology, 7th edition. GL Wied, CM Keebler, LG Koss, SF Patten, DL Rosenthal, eds. Tutorials of Cytology, Chicago, 1992, pp. 302–306.

Murphy WM, Beckwith JB, Farrow GM: Tumors of the kidney, bladder, and related urinary structures in Atlas of Tumor Pathology, 3rd series, Fascicle 11. Armed Forces Institute of Pathology, Washington, DC, 1994, pp. 193–297.

Nabi G, Greene D, O'Donnell MO. Suspicious urinary cytology with negative evaluation for malignancy in the diagnostic investigation of haematuria: how to follow up? J Clin Pathol 2004; 57:365–8.

Wiener HG, Vooijs GP, and van't Hof-Grootenboer B: Accuracy of urinary cytology in the diagnosis of primary and recurrent bladder cancer. Acta Cytol 1993; 37: 163–169.

7
Specimen Collection and Processing

Not to be minimized is the quality of the specimen submitted for microscopic examination. Each laboratory must decide on the best way to collect and process specimens, considering the demands of the clinical setting, ease of preparation, and expense.

Collection

Patients should be instructed to empty their bladders before beginning the collection process. Hydration over a 2–3 hour period after the initial morning voiding (which is discarded) can produce a high volume, good quality specimen, if processing is prompt. A minimal volume of 25 ml is recommended. Some people advocate that the patient jump up-and-down to facilitate increased exfoliation of cells. Collection of samples over a prolonged period, e.g., 24-hours, results in a useless specimen, as the cells will rapidly deteriorate in the toxic urine. Such instructions should be readily available in clinics and on wards so that optimum specimens are received in the cytology laboratory.

While these authors acknowledge that catheterization bears some risk for infection, the value of obtaining a fresh catheterized specimen, especially from females, far outweighs the risk of a urinary tract infection if the catheterization procedure is carefully performed.

Finally, if urinary cytology is to be diagnostic, samples obtained by irrigation (washings) are definitely preferred over voided urines from patients in whom a neoplasm is suspected, either clinically or based on previous urine cytologies. The difference between a well obtained, freshly prepared bladder washing, and a spontaneously voided urine sample is considerable (Figs. 7.1, 7.2). In fact, the authors consider it imprudent to make a "positive" diagnosis on a voided urine unless the changes are so dramatically high grade and unequivocal that a novice could make the call. On the other hand, reliable diagnoses can be made on irrigation specimens from the upper tract, including the low grade lesions, if cells are abundant and well preserved.

Processing

"Freshness" is the key to obtaining a urinary tract sample sufficient for a definitive diagnosis. Rapid processing of unfixed specimens is mandatory. If the clinical setting does not permit immediate processing of fresh specimens, then methods should be provided for immediate fixation. Farrow advocates use of twice the volume of 70% ethyl alcohol to one volume of urine with refrigeration if possible. No more than 8 hours should elapse before the specimen is processed. Carbowax fixation (Saccomanno fixative) is also an effective means of preserving cellular criteria when fresh specimens are unfeasible. Fluids used in processing liquid-based Pap tests are also useful in preserving urines for a short period of time. If specimens must be prefixed, fixation artifact and various changes produced by the technique should be considered when choosing an appropriate procedure.

Whether one chooses to utilize membrane filters, cytocentrifugation, or any combination of procedures, cell loss and optimal staining should be carefully controlled. Processing by the two FDA approved methods for liquid-based Pap tests is gaining in popularity. The least effective method is to smear the centrifuged sediment, as cells tend to float to the top of the fixative line, with loss of much of the sediment. Bloody urines should be pre-treated to lyse the blood to enable contemporary processing techniques and remove potentially obscuring red cells.

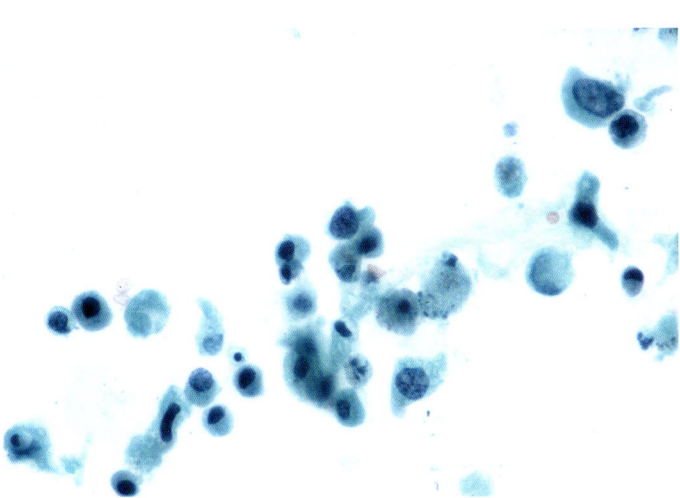

FIGURE 7.1. High Grade Urothelial Carcinoma—voided urine: Most of the cells are enlarged, but are also severely degenerated. Only a few have sufficient cellular preservation on which to confidently base the diagnosis. (400x)

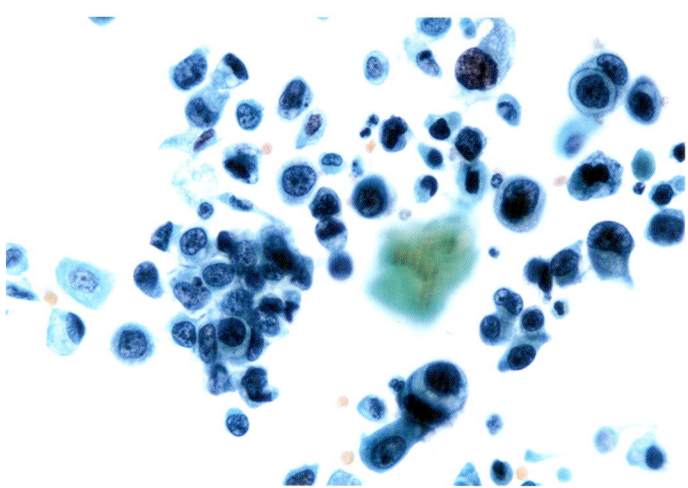

FIGURE 7.2. High Grade Urothelial Carcinoma—bladder washing: An irrigated sample from the same patient whose specimen is displayed in Fig. 7.1. Note the improved cellular preservation by the fresh collection. A tissue equivalent diagnosis can be made. (400x)

Suggested Reading

Bales CE: A semi-automated method for preparation of urine sediment for cytologic evaluation. Acta Cytol 1981; 25:323–326.

Koss LG, Deitch D, Ramanathan R, and Sherman AB: Diagnostic value of cytology of voided urine. Acta Cytol 1985; 29:810–816.

Murphy WM, Crabtree WN, Jukkola AF, and Soloway MS: The diagnostic value of urine versus bladder washing in patients with bladder cancer. J Urol 1981; 126:320–322.

Pearson JC, Kromhout L, and King EB: Evaluation of collection and preservation techniques for urinary cytology. Acta Cytol 1981; 25:327.

Trott PA, and Edwards L: Comparison of bladder washings and urine cytology in the diagnosis of bladder cancer. J Urol 1973; 110:664.

Index

Accuracy of urinary cytology, 166
Acute inflammatory cells, 38
  catheter sample, 39
  herpes simplex infections, 44
  high-grade urothelial carcinomas, 104, 105
  non-viral inclusions, 52, 53
  voided urine, 17
Adenocarcinoma
  atypical glandular cells versus, 5–6
  differential diagnosis of glandular cells in urine, 150
  high-grade urothelial carcinoma versus, 63, 99
Aging/elderly, inclusions, 52, 53
Architecture/organization, *see also* Cellularity; Nuclear crowding/overlap
  high-grade papillary carcinomas, 88
  low-grade papillary carcinomas, 69, 72, 74, 75, 77–79
  morphologic differences, sample collection method and, 21
  progressive cytological changes, 60

Atypias
  assessment of, 7
  drug-induced, 22, 66, 122, 123, 131–140
  flat lesions with, 58
  glandular cells versus adenocarcinoma, 5–7
  indeterminate and low malignant potential, 20, 22, 29, 37, 55, 59, 68
  indeterminate for neoplasia, 22, 29, 37, 55, 59
  mild-to-moderate, 80
  minimal, with low-grade lesions, 72
  radiation-induced, 124, 141–145
  reactive, *see* Inflammation/inflammatory cells/reactive atypias
  of unknown significance, 58, 59

Bacillus Calmette-Guerin, 122–123, 131–135
Background, *see also* Cell fragments
  carcinoma in situ, 65
  comparison of major categories of conditions, 20

175

Background (*cont.*)
  high-grade urothelial
      carcinomas, 94, 104–107
    diagnostic tumor cells and,
        107
    invasion, indicators of, 106
  mimics of high-grade lesions,
      66
  mimics of low-grade lesions, 62
Bacteria, 17, 39
Basal cells, normal, 31, 32
Basal layers, 6, 21
Basement membrane, 6
Benign conditions
  atypia, indeterminate, 29, 55
  casts, 49–51
  crystals, 54
  hemangioma, renal pelvis, 67
  low-grade lesions versus, 59, 60
  normal cells, 25, 30–33
    bladder washing and, 32
    catheter sample, 13, 14, 26
    instrumentation artifact, 20
    voided sample, 16
  reactive cell changes, 21–28,
      34–36, 38–41
    bladder washing sample, 23,
        34–36, 38, 40, 41
    catheter sample, 24–28, 39
    nonviral inclusions, 52, 53
    viral infections, 42–47
  tubular epithelial cells, 48
Biopsy
  low-grade papillary carcinoma,
      69, 86
  high grade papillary carcinoma,
      88, 89
Bladder, 5
  condyloma, 47
  differential diagnosis of
      glandular cells in urine,
      150
  sample collection
    catheter, *see* Catheter samples
    washing/irrigation, *see*
        Washing/irrigation samples
  uncommon lesions, 149,
      152–162
Bladder mapping, 64
Blood/hematuria
  erythrocyte casts, 51
  herpes simplex infections, 44
  high-grade urothelial
      carcinomas, 106, 107
  lithiasis/calculus passage and,
      124
  presentation with, 150
  pre-treatment of urine
      specimens, 170
  sample collection methods and,
      20
Brunn's nests, 5
Busulfan, 123

Calculus disease/lithiasis, 22, 124,
    147
  and cancer incidence, 124
  mimics of high-grade lesions,
      66
  mimics of low-grade lesions, 62
Calyces, 5, 6
Carbowax fixative, 170
Carcinoma in situ, 58, 59, 63–65,
    90, 91, 171, 172
Casts, 22, 49–51
Catheter samples
  instrumentation artifact, 65
  morphologic differences,
      sample collection method
      and, 20, 21
  normal reactive conditions, 9,
      24–28, 39
  specimen collection, 169
  women, presentation with
      hematuria and, 150–151
Cell clusters, normal conditions, 9,
    25, 26
Cell debris, *see* Background; Cell
    fragments
Cell dissociation, low-grade
    urothelial carcinomas, 84,
    85

Cell fragments, *see also* Background
  high-grade urothelial carcinomas, 96, 97
  instrumentation artifact, 30–32
  morphologic differences, sample collection method and, 21
  normal samples, 31, 32
Cell preservation, 169, 171, 172; *see also* Degeneration
Cell sheets, *see* Tissue fragments/cell sheets
Cell size
  carcinoma in situ, 65
  classification and grading
    high-grade lesions, 62, 63
    low grade/grade II lesions, 61
    progressive cytological changes, 60
  cytological changes, progressive, 60
  drug-induced atypias, 123
  high-grade urothelial carcinomas, 98, 100–103
  classification and grading, 62, 63
  polyoma virus-infected cells, 110–118
  normal, catheter sample, 9, 31, 32
  polyoma virus-infected cells, 43
  radiation-induced atypias, 124
Cell types, morphologic differences, sample collection method and, 21
Cellular casts, 22, 49–51
Cellularity, *see also* Architecture/organization
  carcinoma in situ, 64–65
  comparison of major categories of conditions, 20
  mimics of high-grade lesions, 66
  morphologic differences, sample collection method and, 21
  unsatisfactory sample, 20

Chemotherapy, drug-induced atypias, 22, 122, 123, 131–140
Chromatin, *see also* Hyperchromasia
  classification and grading
    high-grade, 62, 63
    low grade/grade I lesions, 59
    low grade/grade II lesions, 61
    malignant criteria, 62
    mimics of low-grade lesions, 62
    progressive cytological changes, 60
  comparison of major categories of conditions, 20
  high-grade urothelial carcinomas, 66, 100, 101
    versus polyoma virus-infected cells, 102
    polyoma virus-infected cells, 66, 110–118
  low-grade carcinomas, 21, 77, 79
  morphologic differences, sample collection method and, 21
  normal, 8
  polyoma virus-infected cells, 43, 110–116, 118
  reactive/inflammatory changes, 21, 34
  tissue fragments, 96, 97
Classification and grading, *see* Grading/classification of neoplasms
Columnar cells
  enteric, in ileal loops, 121, 125–127
  normal, 6–7, 11
  prostate and accessory sex glands, 5, 6
Concurrent conditions
  calculi and carcinoma, 66
  simultaneous/metachronous tumors, 2

Condyloma, bladder, 47
Connective tissue, basal layer, 6
Crowding, *see* Architecture/organization; Nuclear crowding/overlap
Crystals, 22, 54
Cystic renal cell carcinoma, 150
Cystitis cystica/glandularis, 5, 7, 150; *see also* Inflammation/inflammatory cells/reactive atypias
Cystoscopy, 2, 20
Cytological criteria, carcinoma in situ, 64–65
Cytology-histology correlation, 165–166
Cytomegalovirus, 22, 46
Cytoplasm
  benign/normal cells, 9
    reactive/inflammatory conditions, 21, 25, 35, 40, 41
    umbrella, 6, 8, 30
    urothelial, 13, 14
  classification and grading
    high-grade, 63
    low grade/grade II lesions, 60, 61
    mimics of high-grade lesions, 66
    mimics of low-grade lesions, 62
    progressive cytological changes, 60
  comparison of major categories of conditions, 20
  drug-induced atypias, 123
  high-grade carcinomas
    mimics of, 66
    papillary, 90
    urothelial, 93, 99, 103, 104, 114
    polyoma virus-infected cells, 114, 115
  low-grade urothelial carcinomas, 21, 62, 80, 82, 83
  perinuclear, *see* Perinuclear cytoplasm
  reactive/inflammatory changes, 21, 25, 35, 40, 41
  renal tubular epithelial cells, 48
  virus-infected cells
    cytomegalovirus, 46
    human papillomavirus, 47
    polyoma virus, 114
Cytoplasmic vacuolization
  drug-induced atypias, 123
  high-grade papillary carcinomas, 90
  high-grade urothelial carcinomas, 99
  normal cells, 9
  radiation-induced atypias, 124
Cytoxan, 123

Debris, *see* Background; Cell fragments
Decoy cells, 21, 42–43, 101, 111
Degenerative changes, 24, 38, 40
  catheter sample, 24
  high-grade urothelial carcinomas, 92, 94, 102, 104, 105
  low-grade urothelial carcinomas, 83–85
  non-viral inclusions, 52, 53
  reactive/inflammatory cells, 36
  reactive urothelial cells, 27, 28
  voided samples, 83, 171
Denudation, 64, 165
Detrusor muscle invasion, 58, 65
Diagnostic categories, 19–22
  atypical cells, indeterminate and low malignant potential, 20, 22, 29, 37, 55, 59, 68
  benign cellular changes, normal/reactive, 21–22, 34–36, 38–41

morphologic differences,
    sample collection and,
    20–21, 24–33
nonepithelial elements, 22,
    49–54
report formatting, 19, 20
unsatisfactory sample, 19, 20
Diagnostic yield, 166, 167
Disordered cells, *see*
    Architecture/organization
Dome, bladder, 5, 7
Drug-induced atypias, 22, 66, 122,
    123, 131–140
Dysplasia, histological grading
    system, 59

Ejaculate, 22
Endocervical cells, 150
Endometriosis, 12, 150, 155
Endometrium, 150
Enteric cells
    ileal loop and artificial bladders,
        121–122, 125–130
    morphologic differences,
        sample collection method
        and, 21
Erythrocyte casts, 51
Ethanol fixation, 170

Fiber cells, 65, 108, 109
Filling defect, 2
Fixatives, 170
Flat hyperplasia, 58
Flat lesions, 58, 59
Flat lesions with atypia, 58
Formatting report, 19, 20
Fragments, cell, *see* Background;
    Cell fragments
Fragments, tissue, *see* Tissue
    fragments/cell sheets

Genital tract contaminants, 17, 20,
    22, 150
    papilloma virus-infected cells,
        47
    squamous cells, sources of, 7

Glandular cells
    atypical, adenocarcinoma
        versus, 5–7
    classification and grading, 62, 63
    differential diagnosis, 150
    endometrial, in bladder
        washing, 12
    endometriosis, 12, 155
    inflammation and, 5
    normal, 11
    ovarian cancer, 158–162
    prostatic duct carcinoma, 156,
        157
Grading/classification of
    neoplasms, 57–120
    carcinoma in situ, 63–65,
        88–91, 171, 172
    diagnostic yield of urinary
        cytology, 166–167
    high-grade, 59, 60, 62–63,
        88–105, 171, 172
    invasive, 65, 106–109
    mimics of, 65–66, 110–118
    histological grading system, 59
    low-grade
        grade I, 59, 60, 68–72
        grade II, 59, 60–62, 73–87
    progressive cytological changes,
        60
    systems and terminology, 57–59
Grooves, nuclear, 75–77, 82
Ground-glass nucleus, 42, 43,
    110–112, 115, 116, 118
Growth pattern, *see also*
    Architecture/organization
    carcinoma in situ, 64, 65
    high-grade, malignant criteria,
        62
    low grade/grade II lesions, 61
    progressive cytological changes,
        60
Gynecological disorders, 12,
    150–151, 155, 158–162

Herpes simplex virus infection,
    21–22, 44–45

High-grade intraurothelial
 neoplasia (carcinoma in
 situ), 58–60, 62–65,
 88–105, 171, 172
High-grade neoplasms
 classification and grading,
  62–63, 88–105
  histological grading system,
   59
  invasive lesions, 59, 65,
   106–107
  mimics of, 65, 66
  progressive cytological
   changes, 60
  sessile lesions, 57
  WHO-ISUP, 58
 comparative features, 20
 papillary carcinoma, 59
 papillary urothelial carcinoma,
  69, 72–75, 88, 89
 with polyoma virus infection,
  110–118
 urothelial carcinoma, 88–118
  bladder washing sample,
   172
  invasive, 106–109
  voided urine sample, 171
Histiocytes/macrophages, 48, 121,
 127, 150
Histology
 grading system, 59
 correlation with cytology,
  165–166
Honeycomb, 59, 60
Human papillomavirus, 22, 47
Hydration for specimen collection,
 169
Hyperchromasia
 carcinoma in situ, 64
 drug-induced atypias, 123
 high-grade carcinomas, 89,
  90
  papillary, 89
  urothelial, 95, 102–105
 lithiasis/calculus passage and,
  124

low-grade urothelial
 carcinomas, 70, 71, 81
 ureteral, 87
polyoma-infected cells, 42, 43,
 110
radiation-induced atypias, 124,
 142
reactive/inflammatory changes,
 27, 28, 36, 38–40
Hyperplasia, *see also* Inflamma-
  tion/inflammatory
  cells/reactive atypias
 classification, WHO/ISUP, 58
 cytological changes,
  progressive, 60
 flat, 58
 versus low-grade papillary
  lesions, 3
 renal pelvis brushing, 67
 surface cells, columnar
  appearance, 7
 upper urinary tract, 67
Hypochromasia, low-grade
 urothelial carcinomas,
 80–82

Ileal loop/neobladder
 enteric cell appearance,
  121–122, 125–127
 morphologic differences,
  sample collection method
  and, 21
 recurrence in, 128–130
Inclusions, 22
 non-viral, 52, 53
 viral, *see specific viruses*
Indeterminate category, 20, 22, 29,
 37, 55, 59
Infections, 21–22, 42–47
Inflammation/inflammatory
 cells/reactive atypias, 21,
 22
 atypias, assessment of, 7
 BCG and, 122–123, 131–135
 benign/reactive changes, 21–22,
  34–36, 38–41

bladder washing sample, 23, 34–36
catheter sample, 9
classification, WHO/ISUP, 58
comparative features, 20
high-grade urothelial carcinomas, 95, 103–107
histological grading system, 59
hyperplasia, *see* Hyperplasia
invasion, indicators of, 65, 106
lithiasis/calculus passage and, 124, 147
mimics of high-grade lesions, 66
non-viral inclusions, 52, 53
radiation-induced, 124. 141–146
voided urine, 17
Instrumentation artifacts, 20, 24–29
carcinoma in situ, 65
tissue fragments/cell sheets, *see* Tissue fragments/cell sheets
International Society of Urologic Pathologists (ISUP) classification, 58, 59
Invasive neoplasms, 106–109
classification and grading, 57–59
high-grade urothelial carcinomas, 65
indicators of invasion, 65, 106
presentation with, 2
Inverted papilloma, 58
Irrigation specimen, *see* Washing/irrigation samples

Karyorrhexis, 123
Keratinization, 93, 152, 153
Kidney, 5, 48, 67
casts, 22, 49–51
epithelial cells, 22, 48
hemangioma, 67
lithiasis, 22, 62, 66, 124, 147
uncommon lesions, 149–150
Koilocytes, 22, 47

Lamina propria invasion, 58
Liquid-based Pap test, 170
Lithiasis, 22, 62, 66, 124, 147
Loop sample, 21, 121, 122, 125–130
Lower urinary tract, 5
Low-grade neoplasms
classification and grading, 58–62
grade I, 59, 60, 67–74
grade II, 59, 60–62, 73–87
histological grading system, 59
papillary carcinomas, 68, 69, 72–75, 77–79
progressive cytological features, 59
WHO/ISUP, 58

comparative features, 20
hyperplasia, 58, 67
mild-to-moderate atypia, 80–82
reactive hyperplasia versus, 3
ureteral, 86, 87
Low malignant potential (LMP), 22, 37, 58, 59, 68
Lubricant, 33
sample collection method and, 21, 23

Macrophages/histiocytes, 48, 121, 127, 150
Mapping, bladder, 64
Medications, drug-induced atypias, 22, 66, 122, 123, 131–140
Metaplasias, 93, 99, 149
classification and grading, 62–63
squamous epithelium with, 7
Metastases
presentation with, 2
uncommon lesions, 150–151, 156–162
Mild dysplasia, 22, 58, 59

Mimics of high-grade lesions, 65–66, 110–118
Mimics of low-grade lesions, 62
Mitoses
  carcinoma in situ, 64
  classification and grading
    high-grade lesions, 62, 63
    low grade/grade II lesions, 61
    low-grade papillary carcinoma, 69
    progressive cytological changes, 60
Morphology, sample collection and, 20–21, 24–33, 171, 172
Mucin stain, 63
Mucosal fields, ureters, 6
Multinuclear cells
  BCG treatment and, 135
  herpes simplex-infected cells, 44, 45
  radiation-induced atypias, 124, 142, 144
  umbrella cells, 10
Muscularis propria invasion, 58, 65

Neobladder, *see* Ileal loop/neobladder
Nephrectomy, 2
Neutrophils, 34, 36, 44, 93–95, 106
Nonepithelial elements, 22, 50–54
Normal cells, 8, 10, 30
  benign/reactive changes, 21–22, 34–36, 38–41
  bladder washing sample, 31, 32
  classification, WHO/ISUP, 58
  comparative features, 20
  differential diagnosis of glandular and squamous cells in urine, 150, 151
  histological grading system, 59
  histology and cytology, 5–7
  morphologic differences, sample collection method and, 21

Nuclear crowding/overlap
  catheter sample, 26, 29
  low-grade lesions
    classification and grading, 59, 60, 72–74, 80–82
    papillary carcinomas, 73, 75, 78, 79
Nuclear grooves, 75–77, 82
Nuclear membrane
  carcinoma in situ, 64
  classification and grading
    high-grade, malignant criteria, 62
    low grade/grade II lesions, 60–62
  cytological changes
    progressive, 60
  high-grade papillary carcinomas, 91
  high-grade urothelial carcinomas, 92, 94, 98, 100–104
  low-grade urothelial carcinomas, 80–82, 85
  reactive urothelial cells, 38
Nuclear shape, polyoma virus-infected cells, 112–115
Nuclear stripping, 13, 94, 104, 105
Nucleoli
  benign cells/normal conditions
    reactive/inflammatory changes, 34, 38
    squamous cells, 16
    umbrella cells, 10, 16, 32
    urothelial cells, 13
  carcinoma in situ, 65
  classification and grading
    high-grade lesions, 62, 63
    low grade/grade I lesions, 59, 60
    low grade/grade II lesions, 61
    mimics of high-grade lesions, 66

mimics of low-grade lesions, 62
progressive cytological changes, 60
comparison of major categories of conditions, 20
drug-induced atypias, 123
high-grade urothelial carcinomas, 95
classification/grading criteria, 62, 63, 66
polyoma virus-infected cells, 112, 115
inflammatory changes versus low-grade carcinoma, 21
low-grade lesions
classification/grading of, 60, 61, 62
papillary carcinomas, 77
urothelial carcinomas, 82
Nucleus
benign conditions/normal cells, 25
basal cells, 31, 32
umbrella cells, 6, 8, 10, 14, 30–32
cell degeneration, benign cells, 24
chromatin, *see* Chromatin
classification and grading
low grade/grade II lesions, 61
mimics of low-grade lesions, 62
progressive cytological changes, 60
comparison of major categories of conditions, 20
drug-induced atypias, 123
high-grade urothelial carcinomas
mimics of, 66
versus polyoma virus-infected cells, 102
polyoma virus-infected cells, 110, 114, 115, 118

hyperchromasia, *see* Hyperchromasia
lithiasis/calculus passage and, 124
low-grade lesions, *see also specific lesions*
minimal atypia, 72
papillary carcinomas, 69, 72, 75
reactive/inflammatory changes, 34
bladder washing sample, 35
urothelial cells, 27, 28
renal tubular epithelial cells, 48, 49
virus-infected cells
cytomegalovirus, 46
herpes simplex virus, 44, 45
polyoma virus, 42, 43, 110–118
Nucleus-cytoplasmic ratio
benign conditions/normal cells, 25
catheter sample, 9
inflammatory cells/reactive conditions, *see* Nucleus-cytoplasmic ratio, reactive-inflammatory changes
urothelial cells, 14
carcinoma in situ, 64, 65
classification and grading
high-grade, 62, 63
low grade/grade II lesions, 60, 61
progressive cytological changes, 60
comparison of major categories of conditions, 20
drug-induced atypias, 123
high-grade lesions
mimics of, 66
papillary carcinomas, 89, 91
urothelial carcinomas, 96–98, 100, 101, 103, 105

Nucleus-cytoplasmic ratio (*cont.*)
  polyoma virus-infected cells, 110, 111, 116
  low-grade lesions, 21, *see also specific lesions*
    papillary carcinomas, 74, 78
    ureteral, 87
  reactive/inflammatory changes, 34, 36, 41
    bladder washing sample, 35
    urothelial cells, 27, 29
  sample collection methods and, 20–21
  tissue fragments, 96, 97
  virus-infected cells
    herpes simplex, 44
    polyoma virus, 43, 110, 116
Nucleus shape
  high-grade urothelial carcinomas, 98, 100, 101
  classification/grading, 62, 63
  polyoma virus-infected cells, 115, 118
  low-grade lesions
    classification/grading, 60
    papillary carcinomas, 75, 77
    urothelial carcinomas, 76
Nucleus size
  classification and grading, 60, 62
  drug-induced atypias, 123
  high-grade urothelial carcinomas, 62, 95, 101, 104
  low-grade lesions
    classification/grading of, 60, 62
    mimics of, 62
    papillary carcinomas, 75, 79
    urothelial carcinomas, 81
  normal cells, catheter sample, 9
  sample collection method and morphologic differences, 21

Ovarian carcinoma, 158–162
Overlap/crowding, *see* Architecture/organization; Nuclear crowding/overlap

Papillary lesions, 2–3
  classification and grading, 57–60
    progressive cytological changes, 60
    WHO/ISUP classification, 58
  diagnostic yield, 166
  high-grade neoplasms, 88–89
  hyperplasia, 58, 67
  low-grade neoplasms, 68, 69, 72–75, 77–79
    grade I, neoplasms of low malignant potential (PUNLMP), 59, 60, 67–72
    grade II, 59, 60–62, 73–87
Pap test, liquid-based, 170
Paraurethral glands, 5
Performance characteristics, 165–167
  correlation between histology and cytology, 165–166
  diagnostic yield, 166–167
Perinuclear region features, 8, 46, 47
Plasma membrane, normal umbrella cells, 6, 8
Polyoma virus infection
  benign conditions, 21, 42, 43
  high-grade urothelial carcinoma versus, 101, 110, 115
  mimics of high-grade lesions, 65, 66, 110–118
  SV-40 immunostaining, 65, 117
Predictive values, 167
Preservation
  cell degeneration, *see* Degeneration
  fixatives, 170
  morphologic differences, sample collection method and, 21
Prostate cancer
  adenocarcinoma, 5–6
  metastases, 150, 156, 157
Prostatic duct carcinoma, 156, 157

Pseudopapillary cell groups, 20, 71
Pyknosis
  drug-induced atypias, 123

Radiation-induced atypias, 124, 141–145
Radiography, 2, 3, 122
Reactive/inflammatory atypias, *see* Hyperplasia; Inflammation/inflammatory cells/reactive atypias
Reconstruction, *see* Ileal loop/neobladder
Rectal cancer metastases, 150
Recurrent cancers, 128–130
Red cell casts, 51
Renal cell carcinoma, 149–150
Renal pelvis, 5, 6
Renal pelvis brushing, 67
Renal pelvis lesions
  criteria for diagnosis, 2–3
  hemangioma, 67
Renal tubular casts, 49
Renal tubule epithelial cells, 22, 48
Report formatting, 19–20
Retrograde ejaculation, 150

Saccomanno fixative, 170
Salt-and-pepper chromatin, 123
Sample collection, *see* Specimen collection and processing
Schistosoma, 22
Seminal vesicles, 22
Sensitivity, specificity, and predictive values of cytology, 167
Sessile lesions
  carcinoma in situ, 64
  classification and grading, 57
  diagnostic yield, 166
Sheets of cells, *see* Tissue fragments/cell sheets
Simple columnar epithelium, 5
Simultaneous/synchronous/metachronus tumors, 2

Skin cells, 151
Specimen collection and processing
  calculus disease, 66
  cellular preservation, 169–172
  collection, 169–172
  and morphological differences, 20–21, 24–33
  processing, 170
Spindle cells, 65, 108, 109
Squamous cell carcinoma
  bladder washing, 152–154
  differential diagnosis of squamous cells in urine, 151
Squamous cells, 7
  carcinoma in situ, 65
  classification and grading, 62–63
  differential diagnosis, 151
  high-grade urothelial carcinomas, 93, 94
  normal/benign
    catheter sample, 9
    voided sample, 10, 15–17
  reactive/inflammatory changes, 36, 41
Squamous differentiation, high-grade urothelial carcinomas, 93
Squamous metaplasia, 151
Stratified epithelium, transitional, 6
Stripped nuclei, 94
Surface cells, normal, 6; *see also* Umbrella cells

Terminology, classification and grading, 57–60
Tissue fragments/cell sheets
  bladder washing sample, 31, 32, 34
  high-grade urothelial carcinomas
    classification criteria, 62
    instrumentation artifacts versus, 96, 97

Tissue fragments/cell sheets (*cont.*)
  low-grade carcinomas
    instrumentation artifacts versus, 31, 32, 34, 62, 74, 78, 79
    papillary, 73, 74, 78
    urothelial, 76
Tissue organization, *see* Architecture/organization
Trichomonads, 21
Trigone, bladder, 5, 7
Twenty-four hour collections, 169

Umbrella cells
  classification and grading
    high-grade, 63
    low grade/grade I lesions, 59, 60, 76
    low grade/grade II lesions, 61
  cytological changes, progressive, 60
  normal, 6, 30
    bladder washing sample, 8, 32
    catheter sample, 9, 14
    voided sample, 10
  sample collection method and morphological differences, 21
Unsatisfactory sample, 19, 20
Unusual/uncommon lesions, 149–163
  bladder, 149, 152–154
  kidney, 149–150
  metastases, 150–151, 156–162
Upper urinary tract lesions, 5
  criteria for diagnosis, 2–3
  low grade/grade II lesions, 61, 62, 86, 87
Urachus, vestigial, 5
Ureters, 2, 5
  ileal loops, access via, 122
  low-grade urothelial carcinomas, 86, 87
  normal, 6
Urethra, 2, 5
  normal, 6
  squamous cells from, 7
Urethral brushing, herpes simplex-infected cells, 45
Urothelial carcinomas, *see* High-grade neoplasms; Low-grade neoplasms
Urothelial cells, *see* Benign conditions
Urothelial sheets, *see* Tissue fragments/cell sheets
Uterine cancer, 150

Vacuolization, cytoplasm, *see* Cytoplasmic vacuolization
Vaginal cell contamination, 7, 15, 17, 20, 47, 150
Vesicular cytoplasm, normal urothelial cells, 8, 30
Vestigial urachus, 5
Voided samples
  bladder irrigation, comparison of samples, 170–172
  casts, 49–51
  collection, 169
  cytomegalovirus-infected cells, 46
  degenerative changes
    high-grade urothelial carcinoma, 92
    and interpretation of specimen, 92
  herpes simplex infections, 44
  morphologic differences, sample collection method and, 20, 21
  non-viral inclusions, 52, 53
  normal cells, 7, 10, 15, 16
  polyoma virus-infected cells, 42, 43
  squamous cells in, 7, 15

Washing/irrigation samples
  atypical cells, indeterminate and low malignant potential, 29, 37, 55, 68

calculus disease, 66
crystals, 54
endometrial cells, 12
high-grade urothelial carcinomas, 91, 93, 94, 96–98, 100, 101, 105
instrumentation artifacts, 20, 24–29, 65; *see also* Tissue fragments/cell sheets
lubricant, 21, 23, 33
mimics of low-grade lesions, 62
morphologic differences, sample collection method and, 20–21
normal cells, 8, 11
  sheets of, 31, 32
  umbrella, 8
  urothelial cells, 23
papillomavirus-infected cells, 47
reactive/inflammatory cells, 34, 36, 38, 41
specimen collection, 170
tissue fragments, 96, 97
voided urine comparison, 170–172
World Health Organization-International Society of Urologic Pathologists (WHO-ISUP) consensus classification, 58, 59